Copyright©2019, Ketoveo. All Rights Reserved.

In no way is it legal to reproduce, duplicate, or transmit any part of this document, in either electronic means or in printed format. Recording of this publication is strictly prohibited and any storage of this document is not allowed unless written permission from the publisher. All rights reserved.

The information provided herein is stated to be truthful and consistent, in that any liability, in terms of inattention or otherwise, by any usage or abuse or any policies, processes, or directions contained within is the solitary and utter responsibility of the recipient reader. Nutritional values have been calculated with due care and attention. However, there may be differences due to the variance of each individual kitchen creation caused by ingredient amounts, brand differences, different cuts and quality of meats, etc. The nutritional values of these recipes are provided as a guideline only. Under no circumstance will any legal responsibility or blame be held against the publisher for any reparation, damages, or monetary loss due to the information herein, either directly or indirectly.

Respective authors own all copyrights not held by the publisher.
The information herein is offered for informational purposes solely, and is universal as so. The presentation of the information is without contract or any type of guarantee assurance.

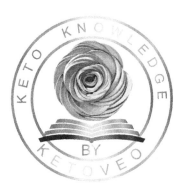

Go to **www.ketoveo.com** for more guides and resources to help you on your keto journey.

Contents

Thai Coconut Soup 8
Chicken Taco Soup 9
Hot Buffalo Chicken Soup 11
Cauliflower Soup 12
Creamy Garlic Chicken Soup 13
Fried Sage with Cauliflower Soup 15
Cream of Zucchini Soup 16
Lemon Chicken Soup 17
Chicken Stew 19
Bacon Cauliflower Chowder 20
Green Curried Cauliflower Soup 21
Zoodle Thai Chicken Soup 23
Ramen with Chicken 24
Chicken Cauliflower Rice Soup 25
Creamy Broccoli Cheddar Soup 27
Beef Shirataki Noodle Soup 28
Chicken Feet Bone Broth 29
Chili Soup 31
Beef Bone Broth 32
Superfood Soup 33
Chorizo Spicy Shrimp Soup 35
No-Cook Chilled Mint Avocado Soup 36
Creamy Cauliflower Soup 37
Avocado Chicken Lime Soup 39
Poached Egg Spring Soup 40
Full Green Soup 41
Sopa De Lima 43
Curried Cauliflower Soup 44
Chicken Mexican Style Soup 45
Creamy Chicken Soup 47

Andouille Sausage Cabbage Soup	48
Pumpkin Cheddar Soup with Chorizo	49
Home Chicken Soup	51
Sausage, Peppers & Spinach Soup	52
Tomato Basil Soup	53
Beef Cabbage Soup	55
Creamy Pumpkin & Sausage Chowder	56
Chipotle Avocado Soup	57
Lamb & Herb Bone Broth	59
Chicken Poblano Soup	60
Easy Chicken Soup	61
Tomato Feta Soup	63
Shirataki Pho	64
Pork & Tomato Soup	65
One-Pot Creamy Meatball Soup	67
Easy Taco Soup	68
Creamy Broccoli & Cheddar Soup	69
Anti-Inflammatory Egg-Drop Soup	71
Ham & Cabbage Soup	72
Creamy Vegetable Soup	73
Roasted Tomato & Garlic Soup	75
Creamy Reuben Soup	76
Chicken Ramen	77
Bacon Cheeseburger Soup	79
Egg-Drop Soup	80
Meatball Zoodle Soup	81
Asian Beef Noodle Soup	83
Creamy Cauliflower & Ham Soup	84
Chicken Fajita Soup	85
Cheesy Cauliflower & Broccoli Soup	87
Chili Dog Soup	88
Crab Soup	89
Asian Meatball Noodle Soup	91

Broccoli Cheese Soup	92
Mushroom Butter Soup	93
Minestrone Chicken Soup	95
Creamy Chicken Bacon Chowder	96
Creamy Mushroom Chicken Soup	97
Turmeric Chicken Soup	99
Queso Chicken Soup	100
Beanless Chili	101
Cream of Wild Mushroom Soup	103
Spicy Chili Con Carne	104
No-Chop Chili	105
Creamy Sausage & Spinach Soup	107
Beef Stew	108
Mussel Chowder	109
Broccoli & Cheese Soup	111
Green Gazpacho	112
Spicy Turkey Soup	113
Beef Stroganoff Soup	115
Wild Mushroom Soup	116
Spicy Pork & Kale Soup	117
Cauliflower Roasted Red Pepper Soup	119
Chicken Soup with Cabbage Noodles	120
Pumpkin & Sausage Soup	121
White Chicken Chili	123
Kale & Spinach Soup	124
Philly Cheesesteak Soup	125
Jalapeño Chili	127
Fennel Vegetable Soup with Celery Root	128
Fish Soup with Aioli & Saffron	129
Cabbage Soup with Chicken Quenelles	131
Crispy Pancetta Cauliflower Soup	132
Goulash Soup	133
Chicken, Egg & Lemon Soup	135

Zuppa Toscana 136

Thai Pork Ribs Soup 137

Broccoli Cheddar Cheese Soup 139

Bacon Cabbage Chuck Roast Stew 140

Southern Potlikker Soup 141

Turkey Soup with Cilantro Butter 143

Asian Meatball Chicken Soup 144

Hamburger Soup 145

Mushroom Soup 147

Cauliflower, Leek & Coconut Cream Soup 148

Creamy Curried Cauliflower Soup 149

Creamy Broccoli & Leek Soup 151

Cream of Mushroom Soup 152

Shiitaki Mushroom, Spinach & Asparagus Soup 153

Beef Noodle Soup with Shiitake Mushrooms & Baby Bok Choy 155

Simple Egg-Drop Soup 156

Bacon, Leek & Cauliflower Soup 157

Creamy Pulled Pork Soup 159

Cheesy Zucchini Soup 160

Simple Coconut Seafood Soup 161

Brazilian Hot Shrimp Soup 163

Creamy Leek & Salmon Soup 164

Salmon Soup 165

Chicken Soup 167

Thai Chicken Broth 168

Enchilada Chicken Soup 169

Cabbage Soup 171

Thai Beef & Broccoli Soup 172

KETO SOUPS COOKBOOK

THAI COCONUT SOUP

Servings: 6

Nutritional Facts Per Serving:
Net Carbs: 3.6 g   Protein: 27 g
Fat: 17 g   Calories: 274 kcal

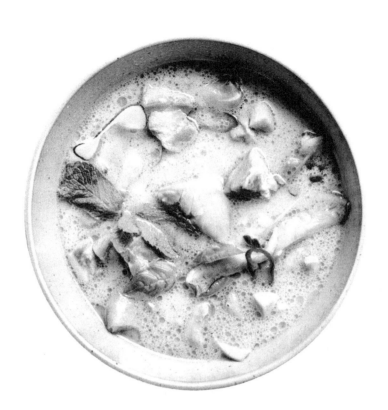

INGREDIENTS

4 chicken breasts, large
14 oz coconut milk
14 oz chicken broth
28 oz filtered water
¼ cup Red Boat fish sauce
2 tbsp Thai garlic chili paste
1 tbsp coconut aminos
1 oz lime juice
1 tsp ground ginger
2 sprigs fresh Thai basil
Cilantro for garnish

This is how you make the recipe

1. Thinly slice chicken breast into ¼-inch thick strips, then cut once more to make them bite-sized.

2. In a large stock pot, combine coconut milk, broth, water, fish sauce, chili sauce, coconut aminos, lime juice, ginger, and basil. Bring to a boil over high heat.

3. Stir in chicken pieces, reduce heat to medium-low, and cover pot; simmer for 30 minutes.

4. Remove basil leaves from the soup and garnish with cilantro.

5. Enjoy!

CHICKEN TACO SOUP

Servings: 8

Nutritional Facts Per Serving:
Net Carbs: 9 g   Protein: 38 g
Fat: 11.75 g   Calories: 304 kcal

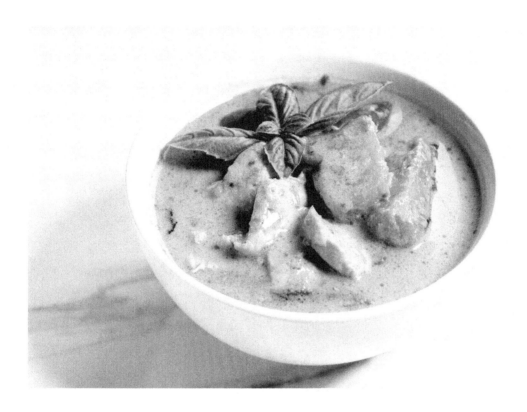

INGREDIENTS

2 lb boneless skinless chicken breasts
16 oz cream cheese
1 (1-oz) package Hidden Valley Original Ranch Seasoning and Salad Dressing Mix
3 tbsp southwestern seasoning
20 oz Ro-tel
4 cups chicken broth

This is how you make the recipe

1. Place all ingredients in a 6 quart slow cooker. Cover and cook on low for 6 to 8 hours.

2. Remove chicken from slow cooker and shred with two forks. Return to slow cooker and stir.

3. Serve with cheese, cilantro and sour cream, if desired.

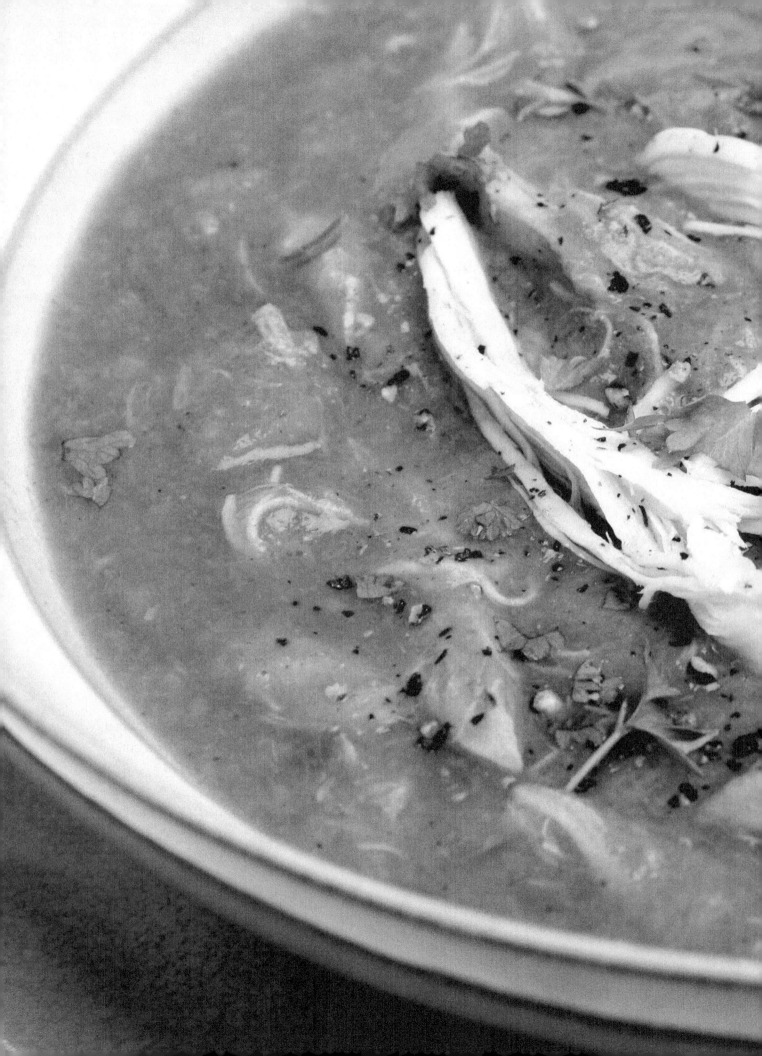

HOT BUFFALO CHICKEN SOUP

Servings: 8

Nutritional Facts Per Serving:
Net Carbs: 13.4 g Protein: 38.3 g
Fat: 13 g Calories: 336.8 kcal

INGREDIENTS

2 lb rotisserie chicken, cooked and shredded
3 tbsp ranch seasoning
1 large head of cauliflower chopped
4 cups chicken stock
2 cups chicken broth
1 cup water
1 lb sliced carrots
6 stalks of celery, sliced
1 medium onion, diced
1 tbsp butter
1 cup buffalo sauce
Chopped green onion and blue cheese crumbles for garnish

This is how you make the recipe

1. Boil cauliflower in stock pot with water, ranch seasoning, chicken broth, and chicken stock until very tender; approximately 10 minutes.

2. While cauliflower is cooking, sauté carrots, celery, and onion with the butter. Cook on medium heat until the onions are translucent and the vegetables are fork tender.

3. Using an immersion blender, blend the cauliflower into a purée in the stock pot. It should blend completely and form a thicker base for the soup. Add the buffalo sauce and stir.

4. Add the celery, carrots, and onion to the stock pot and stir.

5. Stir in chicken and let cook on low for 20-30 minutes.

6. Serve hot with green onion and blue cheese as garnish (optional).

7. Enjoy!

KETO SOUP RECIPES

CAULIFLOWER SOUP

Servings: 8

Nutritional Facts Per Serving:
Net Carbs: 3.7 g   Protein: 1.8 g
Fat: 1.3 g   Calories: 36.6 kcal

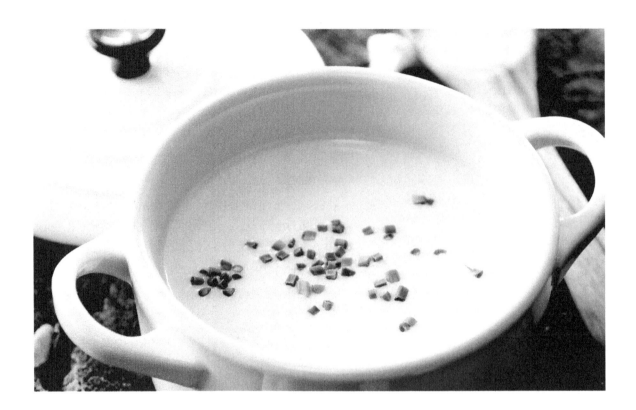

INGREDIENTS

½ tbsp olive oil
2 garlic cloves, minced
1 onion, diced
1 head cauliflower, diced
32 oz vegetable broth
1 tsp sea salt
Fresh grated parmesan cheese and chopped green onion for garnish (optional)

This is how you make the recipe

1. In a Dutch oven (or heavy pot), heat olive oil over medium heat. Add onion and garlic. Cook until softened, about 5 minutes.

2. Add cut up cauliflower and vegetable broth. Bring to a boil then cover and simmer for 15-20 minutes until cauliflower is softened.

3. Carefully pour entire contents of pot into blender. Add salt.

4. Carefully blend until smooth. Serve in bowls with grated parmesan cheese on top and sliced green onions (optional).

5. Serve and enjoy!

CREAMY GARLIC CHICKEN SOUP

Servings: 4

Nutritional Facts Per Serving:
Net Carbs: 2.8 g Protein: 20 g
Fat: 25.8 g Calories: 324 kcal

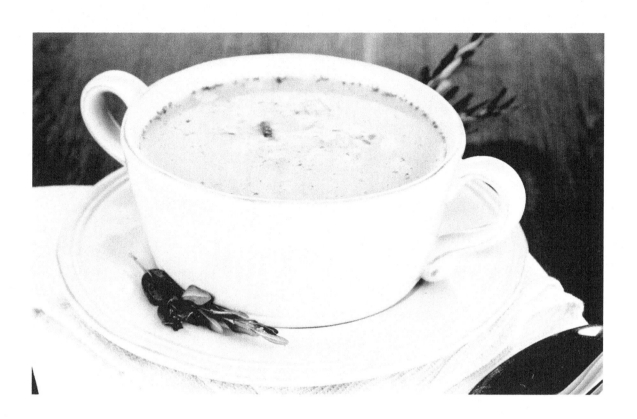

INGREDIENTS

2 tbsp butter
2 cups shredded chicken (1 large chicken breast)
4 oz cream cheese, cubed
2 tbsp garlic seasoning
14 ½ oz chicken broth
½ cup heavy cream
Sea salt to taste

This is how you make the recipe

1. Melt butter in saucepan over medium heat.

2. Add shredded chicken to pan and coat with melted butter.

3. As chicken begins to warm, add cubes of cream cheese and garlic seasoning. Mix to blend ingredients.

4. Once the cream cheese has melted and is evenly distributed, add chicken broth and heavy cream. Bring to a boil, then reduce heat to low and simmer for 3-4 minutes.

5. Add salt to taste and serve.

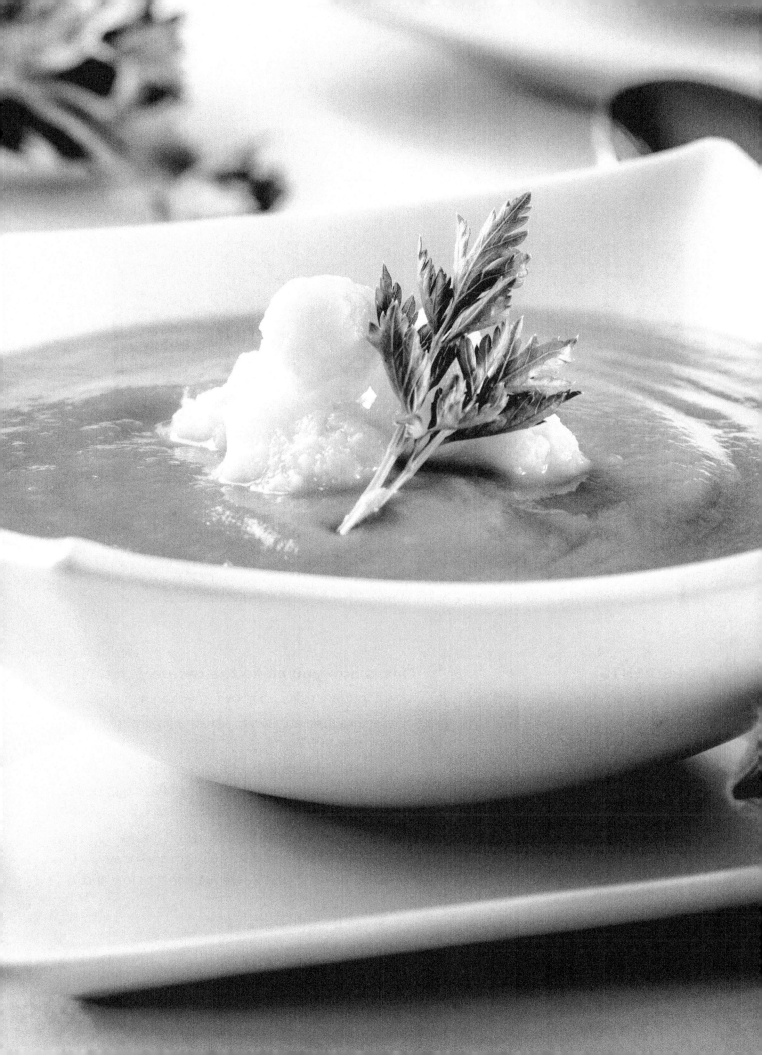

FRIED SAGE WITH CAULIFLOWER SOUP

Servings: 4

Nutritional Facts Per Serving:
Net Carbs: 16.8 g   Protein: 11.5 g
Fat: 53 g   Calories: 584.5 kcal

INGREDIENTS

Large head of cauliflower, cut into florets
5 tbsp of ghee or fat of choice
1 large yellow onion, thinly-sliced
4 cloves of garlic, peeled and thinly-sliced
3 cups chicken stock
1 can full-fat coconut milk
Sea salt and black pepper to taste
For Fried Sage:
1 bunch of sage leaves, separated
¼ cup of lard, ghee or coconut oil

This is how you make the recipe

1. Preheat the oven to 425 °F. Place the cauliflower florets into a large bowl and pour 3 tbsp of ghee, or fat of choice, onto them. Season with salt and pepper, and toss well to coat with fat. Spread cauliflower onto a large baking sheet to form a single layer and place into the oven for 45-50 minutes or until cauliflower florets are golden browned on the edges and tender. Set 4 florets aside for final garnish.

2. Make the fried sage while the cauliflower is roasting in the oven by heating the lard, ghee, or coconut oil in a small skillet over medium heat until hot and add sage (3-4 leaves at a time) and let fry for 4-5 seconds and place on a paper towel to drain, season with salt.

3. Heat remaining 2 tbsp of ghee in a large pot or Dutch oven and add onions and garlic and sauté for 3-4 minutes or until onions begin to soften, add roasted cauliflower, chicken stock and season with salt and pepper. Bring to a boil then reduce heat to low and simmer for 15 minutes, stirring occasionally.

4. Remove from the heat and stir in coconut milk. Then carefully add all of the contents from the pot into a blender as to avoid splashing. Blend until smooth and serve garnished with fried sage leaves and a roasted cauliflower floret.

KETO SOUP RECIPES

CREAM OF ZUCCHINI SOUP

Servings: 4

Nutritional Facts Per Serving:
Net Carbs: 5.4 g   Protein: 4 g
Fat: 2.1 g   Calories: 56.8 kcal

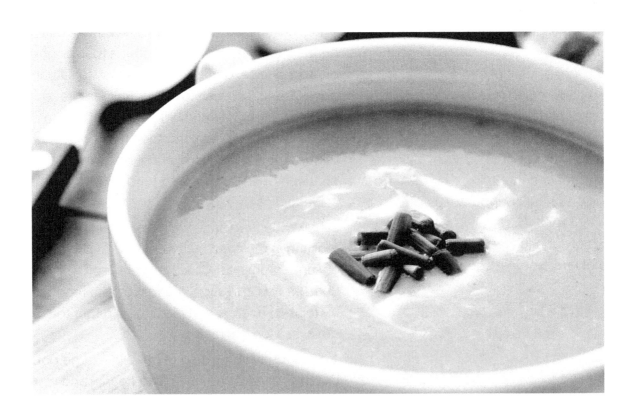

INGREDIENTS

½ small onion, quartered
2 cloves garlic
3 medium zucchini, skin on cut in large chunks
32 oz reduced chicken broth (or vegetable)
2 tbsp full-fat sour cream
Sea salt and black pepper to taste
Fresh grated parmesan cheese for garnish (optional)

This is how you make the recipe

1. Combine chicken broth, onion, garlic and zucchini in a large pot over medium heat and bring to a boil.

2. Lower heat, cover, and simmer until tender, about 20 minutes.

3. Remove from heat and purée with an immersion blender, add the sour cream and purée again until smooth.

4. Taste for salt and pepper adjust to taste, add grated parmesan cheese if desired for topping.

5. Enjoy!

LEMON CHICKEN SOUP

Servings: 8

Nutritional Facts Per Serving:
Net Carbs: 15.4 g   Protein: 14.6 g
Fat: 8.5 g   Calories: 201.3 kcal

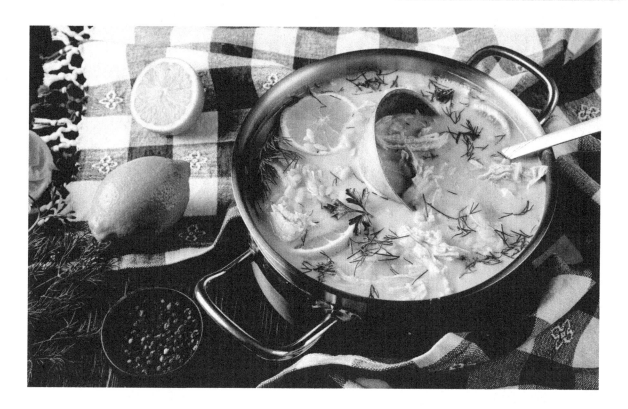

INGREDIENTS

10 cups chicken broth
3 tbsp olive oil
8 cloves garlic, minced
1 sweet onion
1 large lemon, zested
2 boneless skinless chicken breasts
½ tsp crushed red pepper
2 oz crumbled feta
⅓ cup chopped chive
Sea salt and black pepper

This is how you make the recipe

1. Place the olive oil in a large 6-8 quart sauce pot over medium-low heat. Peel the onion. Then quarter it and slice into thin strips. Once the oil is hot, sauté the onion and minced garlic for 3-4 minutes to soften.

2. Add the chicken broth, raw chicken breasts, lemon zest, and crushed red pepper to the pot. Raise the heat to high, cover, and bring to a boil. Once boiling, reduce the heat to medium, then simmer for 5 minutes.

3. Stir in 1 tsp sea salt, and black pepper to taste. Simmer another 5 minutes. Then turn the heat off.

4. Using tongs, remove the two chicken breasts from the pot. Use a fork and the tongs to shred the chicken. Then place it back in the pot. Stir in the crumbled feta cheese and chopped chive. Taste and salt and pepper as needed.

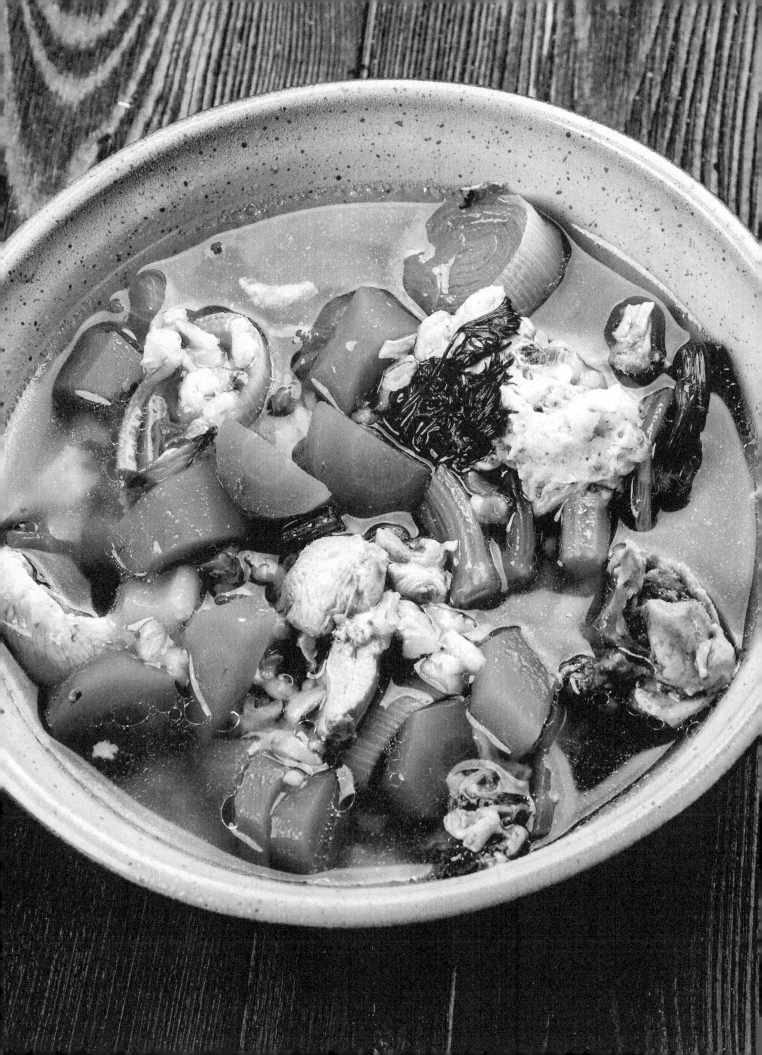

CHICKEN STEW

Servings: 4

Nutritional Facts Per Serving:
Net Carbs: 10.1 g   Protein: 51.5 g
Fat: 39.8 g   Calories: 598.3 kcal

INGREDIENTS

2 cups chicken stock
½ cup carrots, peeled and finely diced
1 cup celery, diced
½ cup onion, diced
28 oz skinless and deboned chicken thighs, diced into 1-inch pieces
1 sprig fresh rosemary or ½ tsp dried rosemary
3 garlic cloves, minced
¼ tsp dried thyme
½ tsp dried oregano
1 cup fresh spinach
½ cup heavy cream
Sea salt and black pepper, to taste
Xanthan gum, to desired thickness starting at ⅛ tsp

This is how you make the recipe

1. Place the chicken stock, carrots, celery, onion, chicken thighs, rosemary, garlic, thyme, and oregano into a 3 quart crockpot or larger. Cook on high for 2 hours or on low for 4 hours.

2. Add salt and pepper, to taste.

3. Stir in spinach and the heavy cream.

4. Sprinkle and thicken with xanthan gum to desired thickness starting at ⅛th tsp Continue to whisk until mixed and cook for another 10 minutes.

5. Serve and Enjoy!

KETO SOUP RECIPES

BACON CAULIFLOWER CHOWDER

Servings: 6-8

Nutritional Facts Per Serving:
Net Carbs: 6.7 g Protein: 4.9 g
Fat: 3.4 g Calories: 82.5 kcal

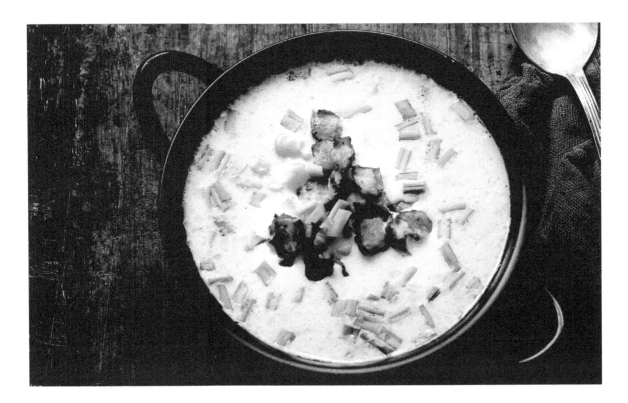

INGREDIENTS

4 slices bacon, cut into 1-inch pieces
1 medium yellow onion, chopped
2 medium carrots, peeled and chopped
2 stalks celery, chopped
Sea salt
Freshly ground black pepper
2 cloves garlic, minced
2 tbsp flour
2 sprigs thyme, stripped and chopped
1 head cauliflower, cut into small florets
4 cups vegetable broth
1 cup whole milk

This is how you make the recipe

1. In a large pot over medium heat, cook bacon until crispy. Transfer to paper towel-lined plate and drain all but 2 tbsp of fat.

2. To pot, add onion, carrots, and celery. Season with salt and pepper. Cook until soft, about 5 minutes. Add garlic and cook until fragrant, 1 minute. Stir in flour and cook 2 minutes more. Add thyme and cauliflower.

3. Pour in broth and milk and bring to a boil. Immediately reduce heat and simmer until cauliflower is fork tender, about 15 minutes. Season with salt and pepper.

4. Garnish with cooked bacon before serving and enjoy!

GREEN CURRIED CAULIFLOWER SOUP

Servings: 4

Nutritional Facts Per Serving:
Net Carbs: 15 g Protein: 11 g
Fat: 22 g Calories: 309 kcal

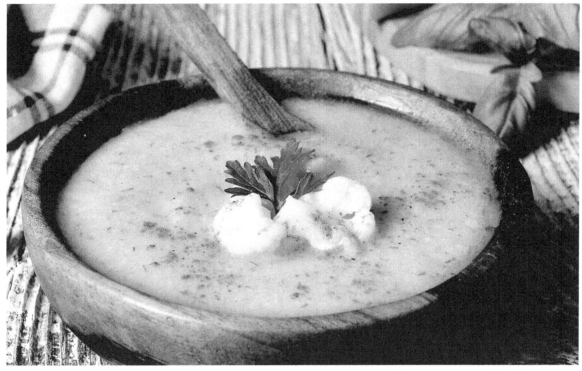

INGREDIENTS

4 cups cauliflower florets, chopped
1 bunch chard, chopped
3 cups baby spinach, chopped
1 small onion
4 cloves of garlic, minced
1 tsp curry powder
4 cups chicken or vegetable broth
2 cups filtered water
½ cup coconut milk
Sea salt and black pepper to taste
2 tbsp ghee, butter, or coconut oil

This is how you make the recipe

1. In small skillet, sauté onion in fat of choice until slightly brown and translucent. Add minced garlic and sauté on low heat for another minute.

2. Add curry powder into skillet and sauté for about a minute, stirring to keep spices from burning (this brings out the flavor of the curry spices).

3. Meanwhile, heat broth and cauliflower in medium soup pot. Simmer, covered, for another 10 minutes.

4. Add chard and water. Simmer covered another 10 minutes.

5. Add spinach and simmer, covered, for another 5 minutes.

6. Turn off heat and stir in coconut milk and add sautéed onions, garlic, and spices.

7. Purée the soup just a tiny bit to make a creamier broth.

8. Salt and pepper to taste.

9. Serve and enjoy!

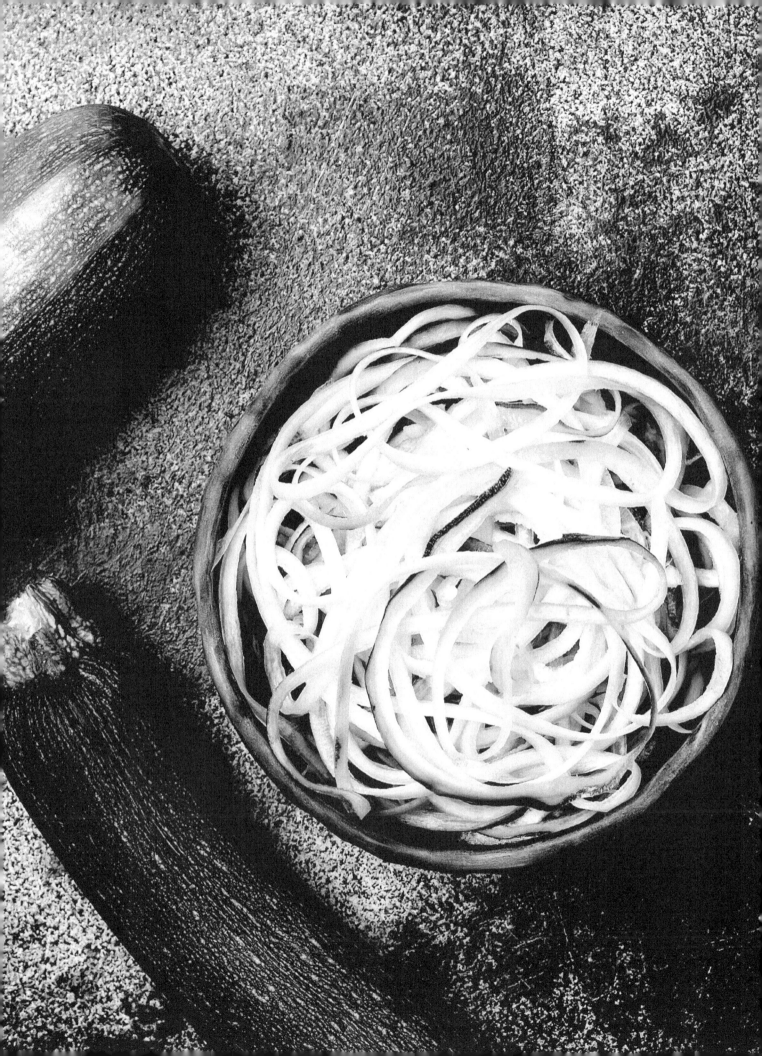

ZOODLE THAI CHICKEN SOUP

Servings: 8

Nutritional Facts Per Serving:
Net Carbs: 6 g Protein: 27 g
Fat: 15.5 g Calories: 268.3 kcal

INGREDIENTS

1 tbsp coconut oil
½ onion, chopped
1 jalapeño, chopped
1 ½ tbsp green curry paste
2 cloves garlic, minced
6 cups chicken bone broth
1 (15- oz) can coconut milk (full-fat)
1 red pepper, thinly-sliced
1 lb chicken breasts or thighs, thinly-sliced against the grain
2 tbsp fish sauce (use Red Boat for paleo)
½ cup chopped cilantro
2 medium zucchini, spiralized
1 lime cut into 8 wedges

This is how you make the recipe

1. In a large sauce pan, heat coconut oil over medium heat until melted and shimmering. Add onions and sauté until just translucent, about 5 minutes.

2. Stir in jalapeño, curry paste and garlic and sauté until fragrant, about 1 minute. Add chicken broth and coconut milk, whisking until fully combined. Bring to a boil, then reduce heat to medium and add red pepper, chicken and fish sauce. Let simmer until chicken is cooked through, about 5 minutes. Stir in cilantro.

3. Divide zoodles among 8 soup bowls and ladle soup over; the heat of the soup will make the zoodles tender. If you are not serving it all at once, only use enough zoodles for each bowl of soup you are serving. The rest will keep well in a covered container for a day.

4. Serve each with a squeeze of lime.

KETO SOUP RECIPES

RAMEN WITH CHICKEN

Servings: 4

Nutritional Facts Per Serving:
Net Carbs: 6.5 g Protein: 13.75 g
Fat: 8.5 g Calories: 156 kcal

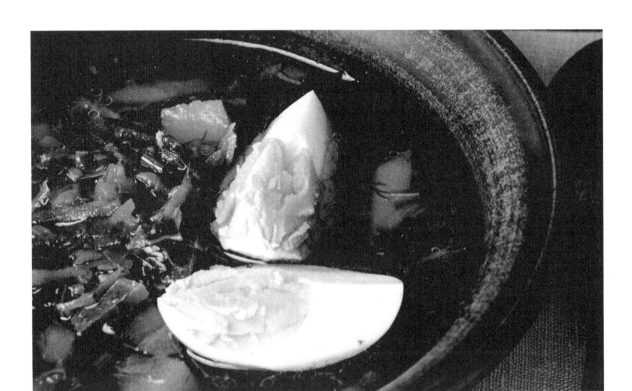

INGREDIENTS

4 cups chicken bone broth
2 knobs of ginger, peeled and sliced thinly
3 tbsp coconut aminos
2 cups thinly-shredded cabbage
2 whole pastured eggs
¼ cup grape tomatoes, quartered (optional)
½ cup cilantro leaves
2 tbsp grass-fed butter or ghee
Sea salt to taste
Pastured cooked meat, such as chicken (optional)

This is how you make the recipe

1. Bring the chicken broth up to a steamy heat and add your ginger. Let steep for 15 minutes, then strain out. Add cabbage to the broth and cook until soft, about 5-8 minutes.

2. While cabbage cooks, heat up a small pot of water over high heat until it reaches a rapid boil. Reduce to a light boil, then carefully add your eggs. Boil eggs for 6 minutes and 30 seconds, then plunge into an ice bath to cool down to room temperature.

3. Stir coconut aminos into your chicken stock. Taste and add more seasonings if desired.

4. Peel your soft boiled eggs and slice in half.

5. Serve keto ramen very hot and top with butter, cilantro, egg halves, meat (if using), and tomatoes.

CHICKEN CAULIFLOWER RICE SOUP

Servings: 6

Nutritional Facts Per Serving:
Net Carbs: 11.1 g   Protein: 13 g
Fat: 23.2 g   Calories: 300.5 kcal

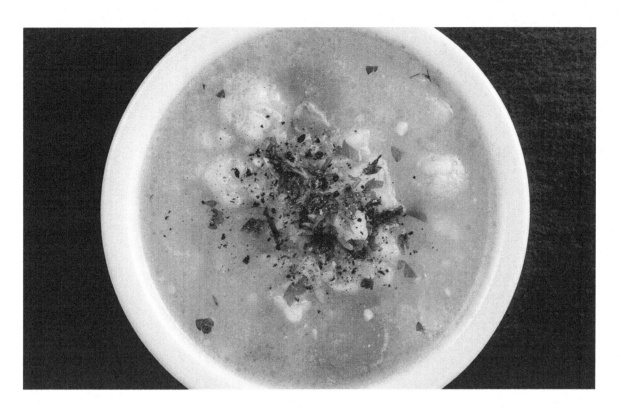

INGREDIENTS

2 tbsp ghee, or olive oil
1 small onion, chopped
2 carrots, peeled and diced
2 stalks celery, diced
Sea salt and black pepper
1 tsp fresh thyme
4 cups chicken stock, or broth
1 bay leaf
1 boneless skinless chicken breast
2 cups cauliflower rice
2 cups canned coconut milk, full-fat
¼ cup fresh flat-leaf parsley

This is how you make the recipe

1. Melt the ghee in a large soup pot. Add the onion, carrot, and celery. Cook for 5-8 minutes, or until the vegetables begin to soften. Season with salt and pepper and stir in the thyme.

2. Pour in the chicken stock and add the bay leaf. Bring to a boil, then reduce to a low simmer. Add the whole chicken breast. Cover and simmer 15 minutes, or until the chicken is cooked through.

3. Remove the chicken from the pot and use two forks to separate it into shreds. Discard the bay leaf.

4. Return the shredded chicken to the pot, along with the cauliflower rice. Simmer 5 minutes, until the cauliflower is cooked. Stir in the coconut milk and parsley and cook until warmed through. Season with salt and pepper to taste.

5. Serve and enjoy!

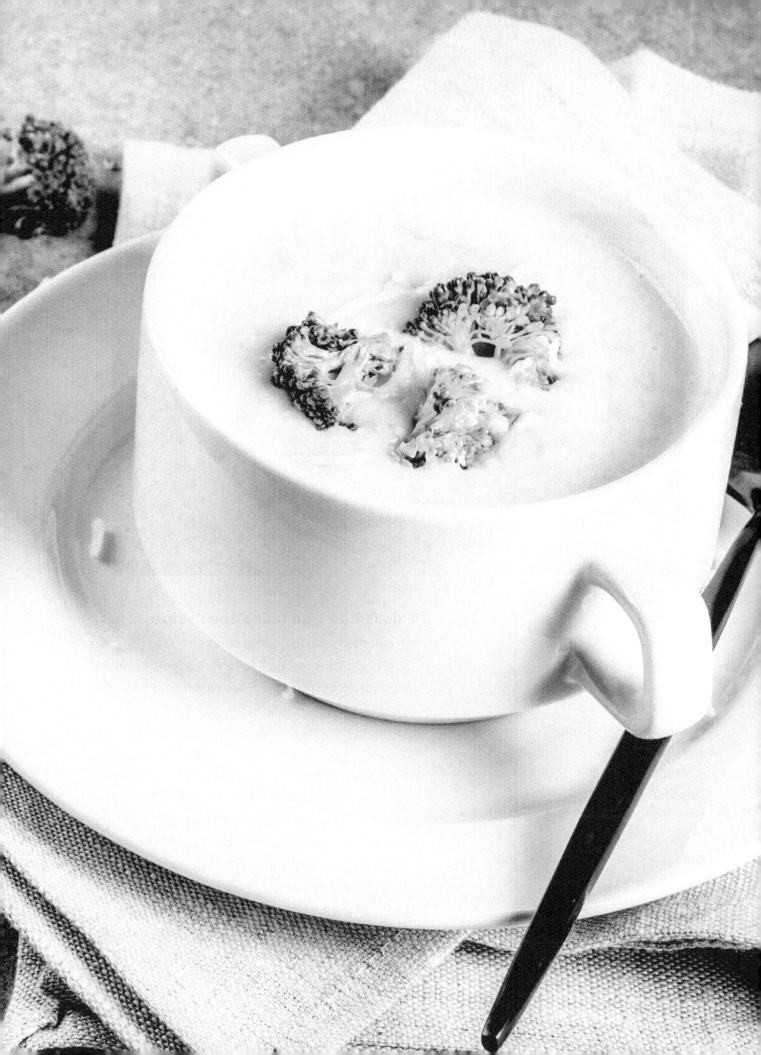

CREAMY BROCCOLI CHEDDAR SOUP

Servings: 4

Nutritional Facts Per Serving:
Net Carbs: 17.4 g Protein: 11.8 g
Fat: 28.8 g Calories: 378.5 kcal

INGREDIENTS

3 tbsp unsalted butter
1 small white or yellow onion, diced
2 cloves garlic, minced
3 tbsp coconut flour
4 cups vegetable broth
2 cups half & half
2 small heads broccoli, cut into florets and stems cut into 1-inch pieces
1 ½ cups sharp white cheddar, grated
Sea salt
Black pepper
Pinch of nutmeg
Greek yogurt or sour cream for garnish (optional)

This is how you make the recipe

1. In a large pot, melt butter over medium-high heat. Add onion and cook until soft, 5 minutes. Add garlic and stir until fragrant, 1 minute. Add coconut flour and cook, stirring constantly, until it turns golden, 3 minutes.

2. Add broth and half & half and bring to a boil. Reduce heat to medium and add broccoli. Simmer until broccoli is bright green, 4 minutes. Then remove four pieces of broccoli (for garnish) and rinse under cold water. Reduce heat to low and cover partially; simmer until broccoli is tender, 15 minutes.

3. If you have an immersion blender, purée soup in pot. Otherwise, working in batches, carefully purée soup in a blender. Pour puréed soup into a large bowl.

4. Immediately whisk in cheddar and season with salt, pepper and nutmeg.

5. Ladle soup into bowls and garnish with Greek yogurt or sour cream (if using), black pepper, and reserved broccoli.

KETO SOUP RECIPES

BEEF SHIRATAKI NOODLE SOUP

Servings: 2

Nutritional Facts Per Serving:
Net Carbs: 6.6 g Protein: 28 g
Fat: 24 g Calories: 360 kcal

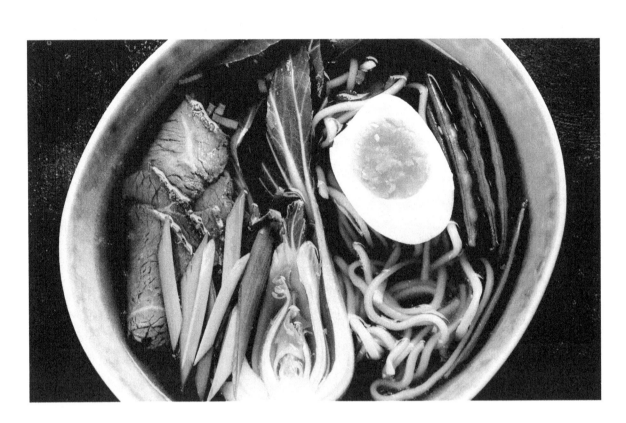

INGREDIENTS

5 oz beef (ground beef, fried minced beef, roast beef, beef meatballs, etc.)
1 tbsp olive oil
3 cups beef or chicken broth
6 oz shirataki noodles
2 garlic cloves minced
1 tbsp fresh ginger, minced
2 scallions sliced
¼ tsp cardamom (optional)
½ tsp sesame oil (optional)
1 hard boiled egg halved
4 leaves bok choy
Water (if needed)
Sea salt and black pepper to taste

This is how you make the recipe

1. Boil one egg in a pot.

2. In the meantime, cook meat the way you prefer such as sautéing ground beef with salt and pepper.

3. In another pot, add bone broth and bring to boil. Lower the temperature, add cooked beef meat, garlic, ginger, cardamom and salt and simmer for 10 minutes.

4. Rinse and drain shirataki noodles and add to the soup. Simmer for another 3 minutes. Add a little bit of sesame oil in for taste (optional). You can add a few bok choy leaves in as well.

5. Divide the soup between 2 bowls, garnish with egg halves and scallions.

6. Serve and enjoy!

CHICKEN FEET BONE BROTH

Servings: 8

Nutritional Facts Per Serving:
- Net Carbs: 1.8 g
- Fat: 5.9 g
- Protein: 10.6 g
- Calories: 104 kcal

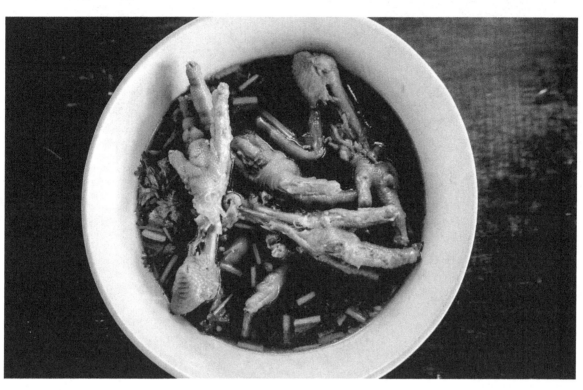

INGREDIENTS

12 pasture raised chicken feet
4 quarts filtered water
1 tsp sea salt
2 tbsp raw apple cider vinegar
1 sprig of rosemary
1 (½ inch) piece of fresh ginger

This is how you make the recipe

1. If your chicken feet still have an outer membrane, you'll need to remove it. In a stock pot, add chicken feet and apple cider vinegar, and fill with water until feet are covered. Bring to a boil, then reduce to a simmer for 10 minutes. Strain and blanch the feet in cold water, allow to cool, then pull off the membranes.

2. Add the chicken feet to a stock pot.

3. Add filtered water until the feet are covered and bring to a boil.

4. Reduce heat to a simmer and skim off any scum that rises to the top with a spoon.

5. Add the ginger, rosemary and salt. Allow to simmer on low heat for 12 or more hours.

6. Remove bone broth from the heat and allow to cool. Strain the liquid into glass jars and serve immediately or chill in the refrigerator.

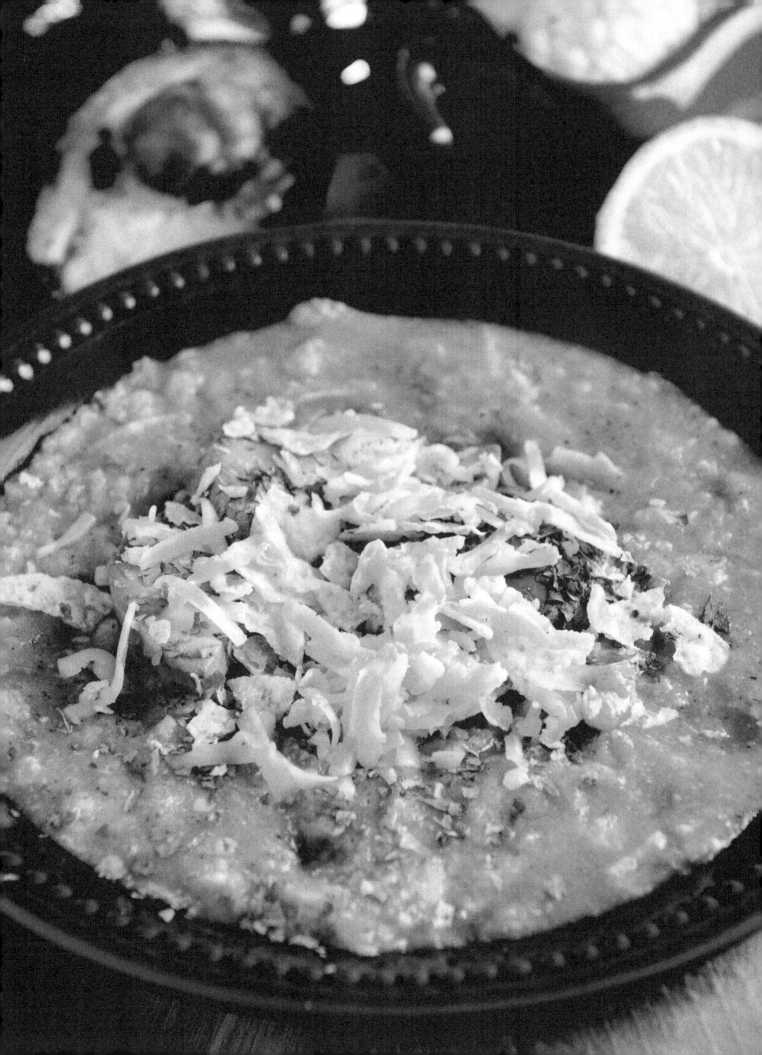

CHILI SOUP

Servings: 8

Nutritional Facts Per Serving:
Net Carbs: 2.5 g Protein: 33.8 g
Fat: 22 g Calories: 354.3 kcal

INGREDIENTS

3 slices bacon, cut into ½-inch strips
¼ medium yellow onion, chopped
2 celery stalks, chopped
1 green bell pepper, chopped
½ cup sliced baby bellas
2 cloves garlic, minced
2 lb ground beef
2 tbsp chili powder
2 tsp ground cumin
2 tsp dried oregano
2 tbsp smoked paprika
Sea salt
Freshly ground black pepper
2 cup beef broth
Sour cream, shredded cheddar, sliced green onions and sliced avocado for garnish

This is how you make the recipe

1. In a large pot over medium heat, cook bacon. When bacon is crisp, remove from pot with a spoon. Add onion, celery, pepper, and mushrooms to pot and cook until soft, 6 minutes. Add garlic and cook 1 minute more.

2. Push vegetables to one side of the pan and add beef. Cook, stirring occasionally, until no pink remains. Drain fat and return to heat.

3. Add chili powder, cumin, oregano, and paprika and season with salt and pepper. Stir to combine and cook 2 minutes more. Add broth and bring to a simmer. Let cook 10 to 15 more minutes, until most of the broth has evaporated.

4. Ladle into bowls and top with sour cream, reserved bacon, cheese, green onions, and avocado.

KETO SOUP RECIPES

BEEF BONE BROTH

Servings: 1

Nutritional Facts Per Serving:
Net Carbs: 1.6 g   Protein: 2.3 g
Fat: 18.6 g   Calories: 189 kcal

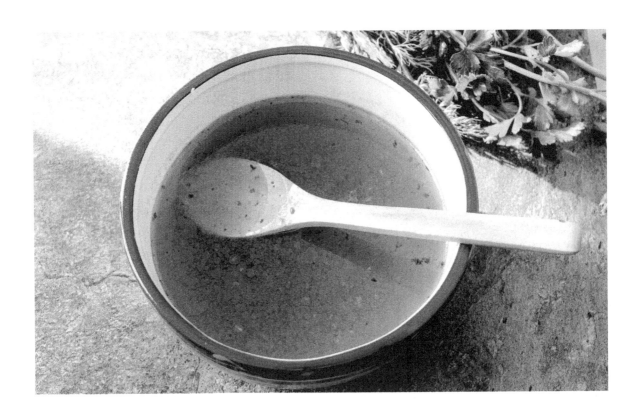

INGREDIENTS

1 cup beef bone broth
½ tsp ground turmeric
¼ tsp sea salt (or more to taste)
1 tbsp grass-fed butter or ghee
Pinch of chili flakes, plus more for garnish (optional)
1-2 tsp seaweed flakes
½ tbsp Brain Octane Oil
Fresh broccoli sprouts for garnish (optional)

This is how you make the recipe

1. Add all ingredients to a small saucepan on medium heat. Bring to a very soft boil.

2. Add all ingredients to a blender and blitz to combine.

3. Pour into a mug and serve warm. Garnish with extra chili flakes and broccoli sprouts.

SUPERFOOD SOUP

Servings: 6

Nutritional Facts Per Serving:
Net Carbs: 7.8 g   Protein: 5.8 g
Fat: 31.5 g   Calories: 334.2 kcal

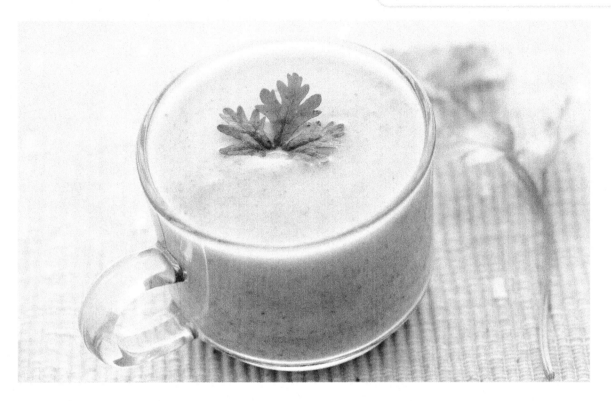

INGREDIENTS

1 medium head cauliflower
1 medium white onion
2 cloves garlic
1 bay leaf, crumbled
½ cup watercress
1 cup fresh spinach
4 cups vegetable stock, bone broth or chicken stock
1 cup cream or coconut milk + 6 tbsp for garnish
¼ cup ghee or coconut oil
Sea salt and black pepper to taste
Fresh herbs such as parsley or chives for garnish (optional)

This is how you make the recipe

1. Peel and finely dice the onion and garlic. Place in a soup pot or a Dutch oven greased with ghee and cook over a medium-high heat until slightly browned.

2. Wash the spinach and watercress and set aside.

3. Cut the cauliflower into small florets and place in the pot with browned onion. Add crumbled bay leaf. Cook for about 5 minutes and mix frequently.

4. Add the spinach and watercress and cook until wilted for just about 2-3 minutes.

5. Pour in the vegetable stock and bring to a boil. Cook until the cauliflower is crisp-tender and pour in the cream (or coconut milk).

6. Season with salt and pepper. Take off the heat and using an immersion blender, pulse until smooth and creamy.

7. Just before serving, drizzle some cream on top and enjoy!

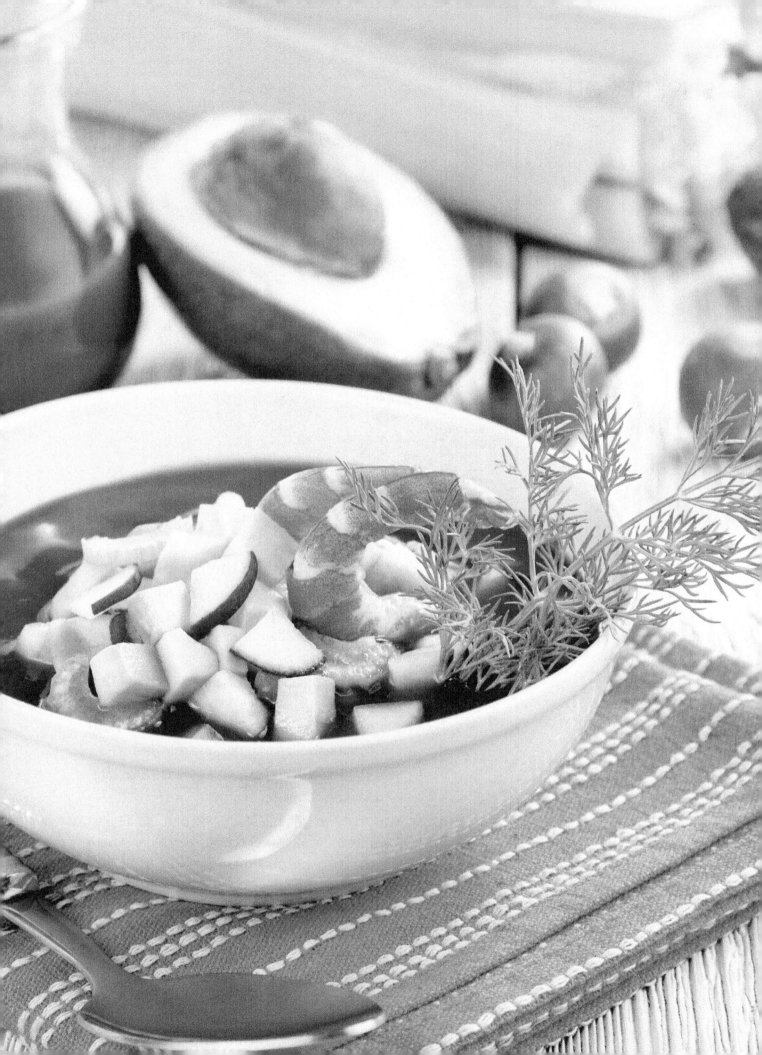

CHORIZO SPICY SHRIMP SOUP

Servings: 6

Nutritional Facts Per Serving:
Net Carbs: 9.2 g   Protein: 34.2 g
Fat: 30.5 g   Calories: 465.3 kcal

INGREDIENTS

1 tbsp + 1 tsp avocado oil, divided
1 medium onion, diced small
3 celery ribs, diced small
1 ripe bell pepper, diced small
4 cloves garlic, sliced
12 oz Spanish-style dry-cured chorizo, diced small
1 tbsp tomato paste
1 ½ tsp smoked paprika
1 tsp ground coriander
1 tsp sea salt
1 28-oz can diced tomatoes
1 qt shrimp or chicken broth
1 lb shrimp, peeled and deveined, chopped
2 tbsp minced fresh cilantro
1 avocado, diced or sliced
Fresh cilantro, chopped for garnish

This is how you make the recipe

1. Heat 1 tbsp of the oil in a large, heavy-bottomed pot over medium-high heat. When the oil is shimmering, add the onion, celery, and bell pepper and cook, stirring occasionally, for 6 to 8 minutes, until the onion is translucent.

2. Add the garlic, three-quarters of the chorizo, tomato paste, smoked paprika, coriander, and salt and cook for 1 minute, stirring constantly, until very fragrant.

3. Add the tomatoes and cook for 5 minutes to cook the raw taste out.

4. Add the broth and bring to a simmer. Cook, uncovered, for 20 minutes.

5. Meanwhile, in a small sauté pan, heat the remaining tsp of oil over high heat. When the oil is hot, add the remaining chorizo and cook for 5 minutes, or until crispy. Set aside to drain on paper towels.

6. Taste the soup and add additional smoked paprika, coriander, and salt as needed. Add the shrimp and simmer until just cooked through, 3 to 4 minutes. Remove from the heat, stir in the minced cilantro.

7. Serve topped with the crispy chorizo, avocado, and chopped cilantro.

KETO SOUP RECIPES

NO-COOK CHILLED MINT AVOCADO SOUP

Servings: 2

Nutritional Facts Per Serving:
Net Carbs: 7.1 g   Protein: 7.5 g
Fat: 35.5 g   Calories: 391 kcal

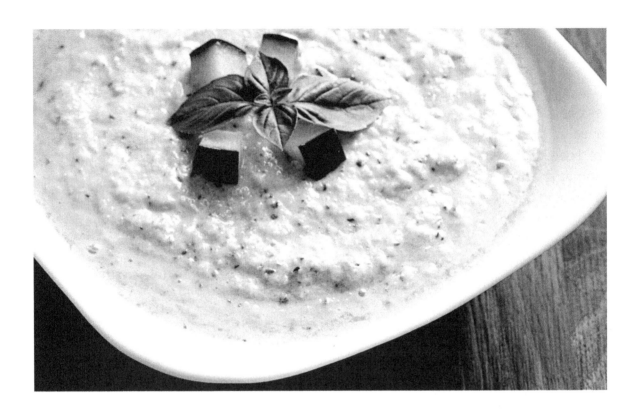

INGREDIENTS

1 medium ripe avocado
2 romaine lettuce leaves
1 cup coconut milk, chilled
1 tbsp lime juice
20 fresh mint leaves
Sea salt to taste

This is how you make the recipe

1. Place all the ingredients into a blender and blend really well. The soup should be thick but not as thick as a purée.

2. Chill in fridge for 5-10 minutes, serve and enjoy!

KETO SOUP RECIPES

CREAMY CAULIFLOWER SOUP

Servings: 6

Nutritional Facts Per Serving:
Net Carbs: 13.5 g   Protein: 6.3 g
Fat: 8.5 g   Calories: 164.7 kcal

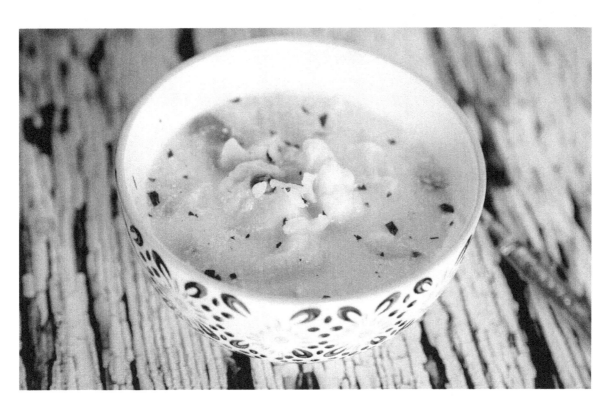

INGREDIENTS

2 tbsp sea salted butter
1 tbsp olive oil
1 large heads cauliflower, cut into small florets
1 white onion, diced
3 stalks celery, sliced
3 carrots, diced
4 cloves garlic, minced
1 tsp dried thyme
1 tsp dried oregano
2 tbsp psyllium husk
2 cups vegetable broth
2 cups milk
Sea salt and black pepper to taste

This is how you make the recipe

1. Heat butter and olive oil in a large pot over medium-high heat. Add in cauliflower, onions, celery, and carrots. Cook for 10 to 12 minutes, stirring occasionally, until vegetables begin to soften.

2. Add the garlic and sauté 1 minute more. Stir in thyme, oregano, and psyllium husk and cook for 1 minute.

3. Pour in the vegetable broth and milk. Stir constantly until the mixture comes to a boil.

4. Reduce the heat to low and simmer 3 to 5 minutes until the soup has thickened. Season with salt and pepper to taste.

5. Serve hot and enjoy!

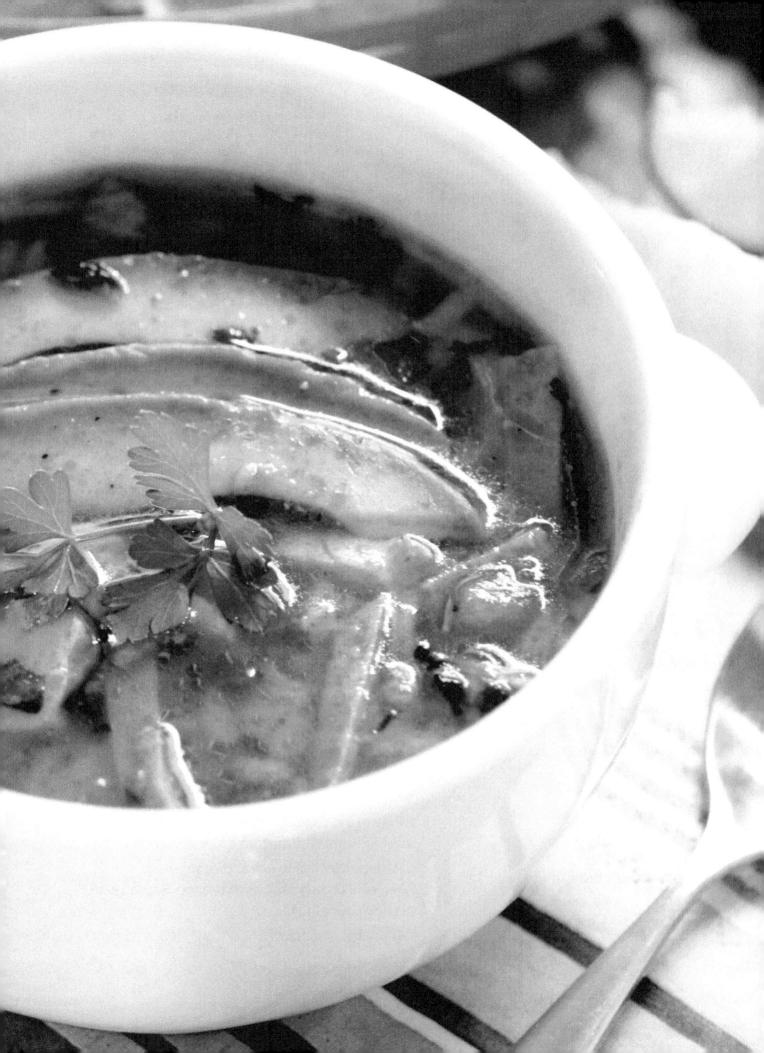

KETO SOUP RECIPES

AVOCADO CHICKEN LIME SOUP

Servings: 6

Nutritional Facts Per Serving:
Net Carbs: 4.1 g Protein: 37.7 g
Fat: 17 g Calories: 339.7 kcal

INGREDIENTS

1 ½ lb boneless skinless chicken breasts*
1 tbsp olive oil
1 cup chopped green onions (including whites, mince the whites)
2 jalapeños, seeded and minced (leave seeds if you want soup spicy, omit if you don't like heat)
2 cloves garlic, minced
4 cans chicken broth
2 Roma tomatoes, seeded and diced
½ tsp ground cumin
Sea salt and freshly ground black pepper
⅓ cup chopped cilantro
3 tbsp fresh lime juice
3 medium avocados, peeled, cored and diced
Cheese and sour cream for serving (optional)

This is how you make the recipe

1. In a large pot heat 1 tbsp olive oil over medium heat. Once hot, add green onions and jalapeños and sauté until tender, about 2 minutes, adding garlic during last 30 seconds of sautéing.

2. Add chicken broth, tomatoes, cumin, season with salt and pepper to taste and add chicken breasts. Bring mixture to a boil over medium-high heat.

3. Then reduce heat to medium, cover with lid and allow to cook, stirring occasionally, until chicken has cooked through 10 - 15 minutes (cook time will vary based on thickness of chicken breasts).

4. Reduce burner to warm heat, remove chicken from pan and let rest on a cutting board 5 minutes, then shred chicken and return to soup. Stir in cilantro and lime juice.

5. Add avocados to soup just before serving (if you don't plan on serving the soup right away, I would recommend adding the avocados to each bowl individually, about ½ an avocado per serving). Serve with cheese and sour cream if desired.

*For thicker chicken breasts, cut breasts in half through the length (thickness) of the breasts, they will cook faster and more evenly.

POACHED EGG SPRING SOUP

Servings: 2

Nutritional Facts Per Serving:
Net Carbs: 6.3 g
Protein: 13.5 g
Fat: 6.5 g
Calories: 154.5 kcal

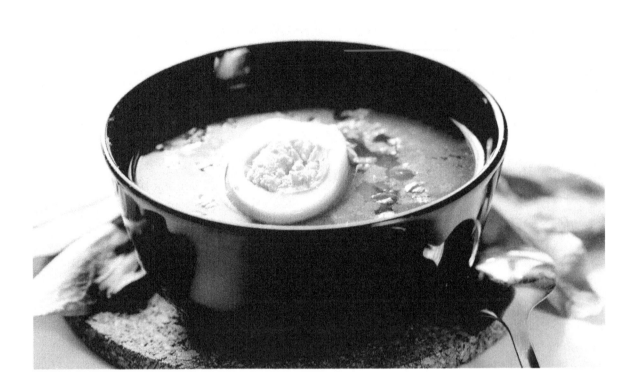

INGREDIENTS

2 eggs
4 cups chicken broth
1 head of romaine lettuce, chopped
Sea salt to taste

This is how you make the recipe

1. Bring the chicken broth to a boil.
2. Turn down the heat and poach the 2 eggs in the broth for 5 minutes (for a slightly-runny egg).
3. Remove the eggs and place each into a bowl.
4. Add the chopped romaine lettuce into the broth and cook for a few minutes until slightly wilted.
5. Serve and Enjoy!

FULL GREEN SOUP

Servings: 6

Nutritional Facts Per Serving:
Net Carbs: 10.3 g   Protein: 9.5 g
Fat: 5.5 g   Calories: 133.5 kcal

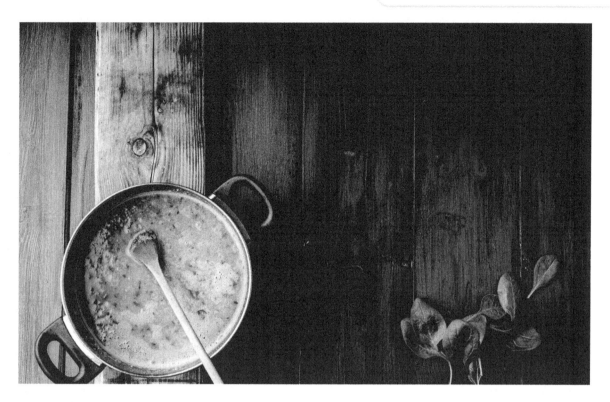

INGREDIENTS

1 medium head of broccoli
1 medium head of cauliflower
3 zucchini
3 leeks
1 brown onion
Sea salt to taste
¼ cup collagen protein
½ cup ghee or butter
1 cup chicken bone broth or filtered water
2-4 garlic cloves (optional)
Fresh or dried herbs - rosemary, basil, thyme, oregano, etc. (optional)

This is how you make the recipe

1. Wash all veggies thoroughly and remove all the dirt from in between the leeks' leaves. Remove the fibrous tops of the leeks.

2. Roughly chop all the veggies and add into a large saucepan.

3. Add remaining ingredients to the saucepan and cook on medium heat until the veggies are soft.

4. If you prefer a beautifully thick and creamy soup, keep the pot simmering so some of the broth can evaporate (1 cup or less remaining). If you prefer a brothy soup, feel free to add additional bone broth if desired.

5. When ready, add all ingredients to a high-powered blender, or blitz the mixture using an immersion blender. Purée until completely smooth and lump free.

6. Taste the mixture and adjust the seasoning as needed, then serve.

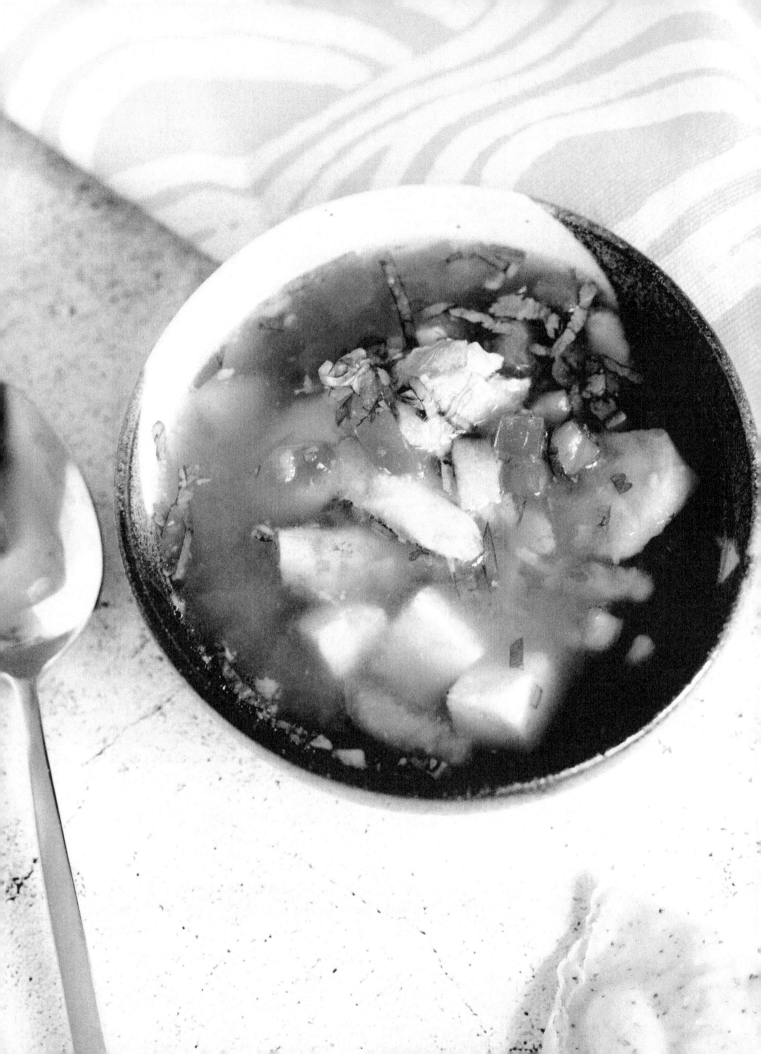

SOPA DE LIMA

Servings: 4

Nutritional Facts Per Serving:
Net Carbs: 8.4 g Protein: 40.8 g
Fat: 13.8 g Calories: 333.8 kcal

INGREDIENTS

4 chicken breast halves
¼ tsp chili powder
¼ tsp garlic powder
4 cups chicken broth
2 serrano chili peppers, cut and scrape out all seeds, chop into small pieces
4 cloves garlic, peeled and minced
2 tomatoes, chopped
½ of an onion, chopped (optional)
1 tbsp olive oil
⅓ lime juice
½ tsp lime zest (optional)
2 tbsp fresh cilantro, chopped
1 avocado, peeled and chopped
Pinch sea salt (optional)

This is how you make the recipe

1. Preheat oven to 400°F, and line or oil a baking dish.

2. Place chicken in dish and sprinkle with chili powder and garlic powder.

3. While chicken is baking, add olive oil to a stock pot on the stove, then saute: minced garlic, serrano peppers, and minced onion for 3 minutes or until veggies are softening.

4. Add chopped tomatoes to the stock pot and simmer for 2 minutes more.

5. Add chicken broth and lime juice to the stock pot and stir, put heat on low.

6. Remove chicken from oven when done, and cool just enough to chop into bite-size pieces.

7. Add chopped chicken to stock pot, and stir.

8. Bring stock pot to a boil, then reduce heat to low, and cover pot with lid.

9. Simmer for 20 minutes.

10. Place some chopped avocado chunks into each individual serving bowl.

11. Pour soup over avocado in serving bowls.

12. Garnish with cilantro.

13. Sea salt to taste (optional).

KETO SOUP RECIPES

CURRIED CAULIFLOWER SOUP

Servings: 6

Nutritional Facts Per Serving:
Net Carbs: 5.1 g Protein: 2.7 g
Fat: 8.5 g Calories: 111.7 kcal

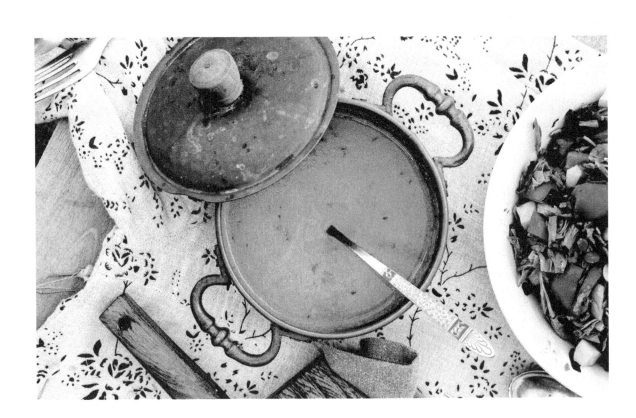

INGREDIENTS

1 medium head of cauliflower
2 ½ cups unsweetened almond milk
⅔ cup unsweetened coconut milk
3 tbsp ghee or coconut oil
½ cup water
1 tbsp curry powder or garam masala
2 tsp powdered ginger
2 tsp garlic powder
2 tsp ground coriander
Pumpkin seeds (optional)
Sea salt & pepper to taste

This is how you make the recipe

1. Combine all ingredients in a medium saucepan. Bring to a simmer and cook, covered, for about 35 minutes or until the cauliflower is completely soft.

2. Purée the soup in a traditional blender, or with an immersion blender right in the pot.

3. Season with salt and pepper to taste. Garnish with pumpkin seeds if desired.

4. Serve and enjoy!

CHICKEN MEXICAN STYLE SOUP

Servings: 6

Nutritional Facts Per Serving:
Net Carbs: 7 g   Protein: 29 g
Fat: 30 g   Calories: 350 kcal

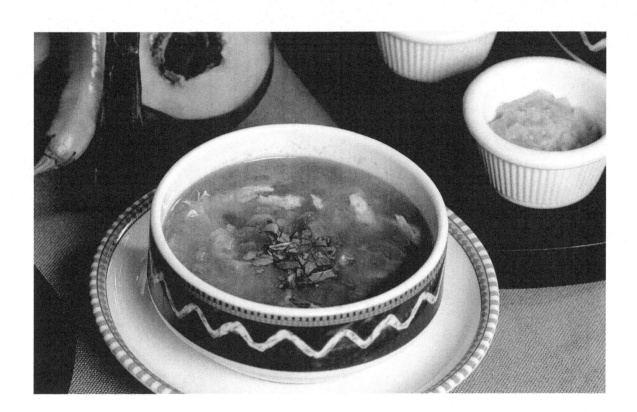

INGREDIENTS

1 tbsp olive oil
1 small onion, diced
2 cloves garlic, minced
1 red bell pepper, chopped
1 tsp cumin
1 tsp chili powder
1 tsp oregano
2 cups chicken broth
1 cup diced tomatoes
½ cup diced green chilies
2 cups cooked chicken
1 cup half and half
4 oz cream cheese
1½ cup cheddar cheese

This is how you make the recipe

1. Heat olive oil in a pot over medium heat. Add onion, garlic, and red pepper, and sauté until onion is translucent (approximately 5 minutes).

2. Add spices. Stir and cook spices for about 1 minute.

3. Add broth, tomatoes, and chilies. Bring to a boil, then reduce heat and simmer 5 minutes.

4. Add remaining ingredients and heat until cream cheese has melted, serve and enjoy!

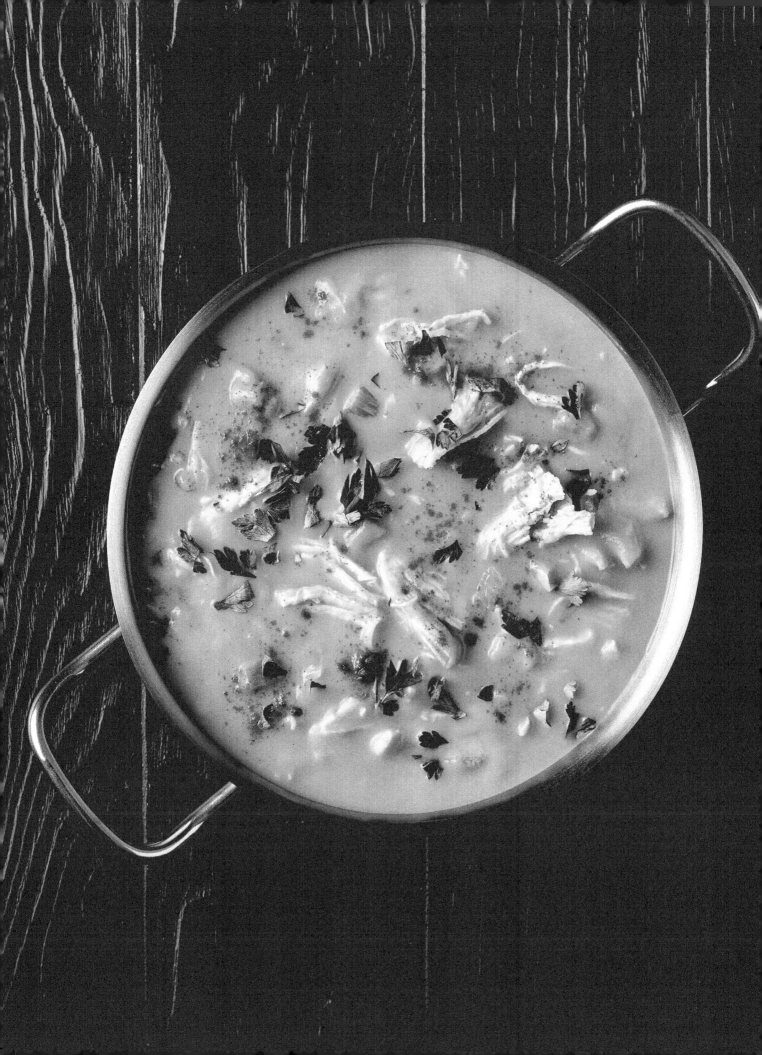

CREAMY CHICKEN SOUP

Servings: 6

Nutritional Facts Per Serving:
Net Carbs: 5 g
Protein: 5.5 g
Fat: 14 g
Calories: 170 kcal

INGREDIENTS

8 ½ cups filtered water
Whole chicken
2 tbsp apple cider vinegar
3 ½ cups cubed fresh pumpkin
Juice from 1 lime
2 tbsp finely chopped ginger
2 medium zucchinis
½ cup fresh parsley, finely chopped
½ cup fresh cilantro, finely chopped
2 tsp ground turmeric
1 cup coconut cream
2 tsp sea salt
2 shallots (optional)
4 cloves of garlic (optional)
1 tsp chili flakes (optional)
Black pepper, to taste

This is how you make the recipe

1. In a slow cooker or stock pot, add chicken and cover with water and apple cider vinegar. (Chicken may remain partially uncovered.)

2. Heat the pot or slow cooker on low heat and simmer for 4 hours, or until chicken can be pulled apart.

3. Carefully remove the chicken from the pot and set aside. Strain bone or skin fragments and reserve the remaining stock. Return stock to the pot and add pumpkin, zucchinis, and ginger. Simmer on low heat for about 15 minutes. Add zucchini and simmer an additional 15 minutes, or until pumpkin and zucchini are tender.

4. While vegetables cook, pull the meat off your chicken and set aside.

5. Once the pumpkin has softened, add the parsley, cilantro, shallots, lime juice, coconut cream and chicken to warm through.

6. Taste the mix and ensure the salt, lime juice and spices are adjusted to your liking.

7. Serve hot, garnished with extra fresh herbs.

KETO SOUP RECIPES

ANDOUILLE SAUSAGE CABBAGE SOUP

Servings: 2

Nutritional Facts Per Serving:
Net Carbs: 39.2 g   Protein: 35.5 g
Fat: 57.5 g   Calories: 848.5 kcal

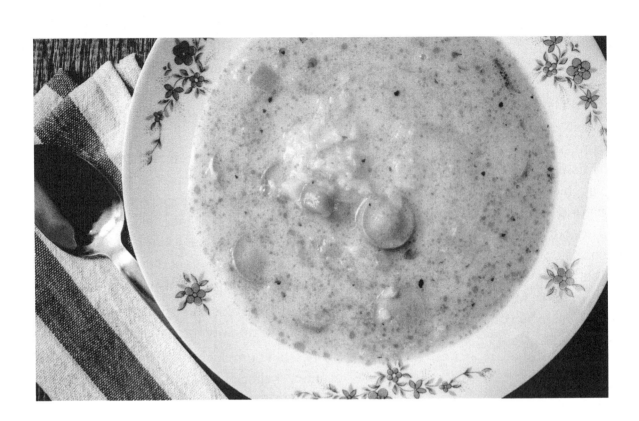

INGREDIENTS

4 links andouille sausage, sliced
1 tbsp olive oil
½ cup shallots, chopped
4 cloves garlic, minced
8 cups cabbage, thinly-sliced
1 cup carrots, chopped
6 cups chicken broth
4 cups water
1 tbsp apple cider vinegar
1 tsp onion powder
1 tsp celery salt
½ tsp dried thyme
1 tsp caraway seeds
1 tsp fennel seeds

This is how you make the recipe

1. Heat the oil in a medium skillet.

2. Cook the sausage with the garlic and shallots until softened and sausage is browned.

3. Add this to the crock pot along with the rest of the ingredients.

4. Cover and cook on high 4 hours or low 8 hours.

5. Serve and enjoy!

KETO SOUP RECIPES

PUMPKIN CHEDDAR SOUP WITH CHORIZO

Servings: 6

Nutritional Facts Per Serving:
Net Carbs: 7.4 g   Protein: 27.2 g
Fat: 39.2 g   Calories: 499.5 kcal

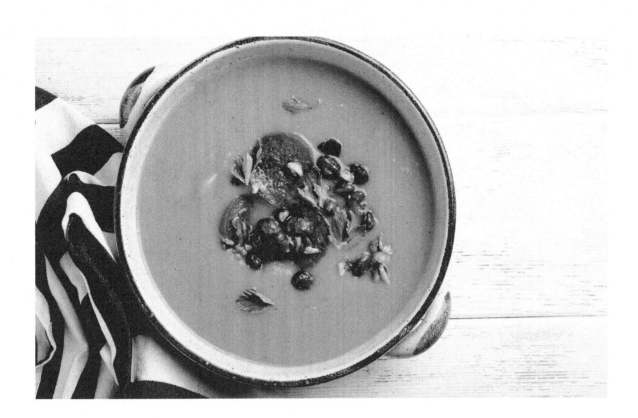

INGREDIENTS

½ onion, minced
15 oz can pumpkin purée
4 cups chicken broth
½ tsp sea salt
½ tsp cumin
½ tsp garlic powder
¼ tsp chipotle powder or more to taste, if you like it spicy
¼ tsp black pepper
6 oz sharp cheddar cheese, grated
1 lb chorizo or other spicy sausage, cooked and crumbled
Sea salt and black pepper to taste

This is how you make the recipe

1. Add onion, pumpkin purée, chicken broth, salt, cumin, garlic powder, chipotle powder and pepper to a large slow cooker. Stir well and cook on low for 4 hours or on high for 2 hours.

2. Add shredded cheese and let melt, then blend soup with an immersion blender or transfer to a large blender or food processor (you may need to work in batches).

3. Spoon into bowls and sprinkle each with chorizo.

4. You can also make this recipe on the stove, in a large saucepan or stockpot. Simply simmer the ingredients from the first step for 20 minutes or so before adding the cheese and blending. Serve and enjoy!

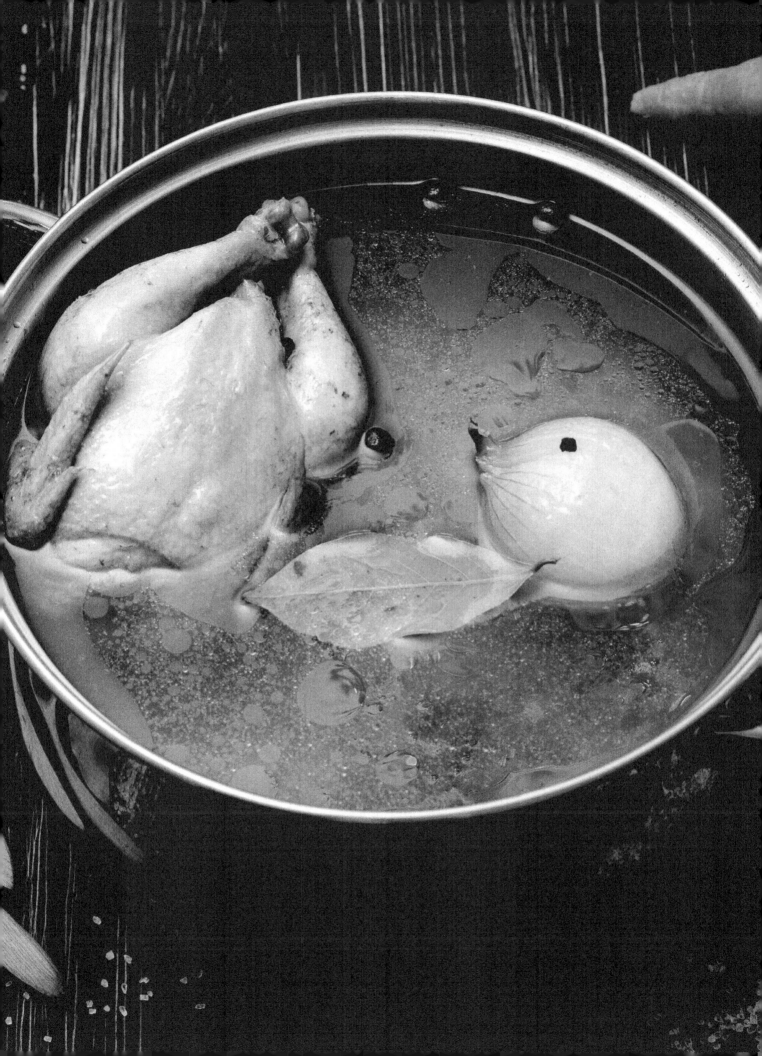

HOME CHICKEN SOUP

Servings: 4-6

Nutritional Facts Per Serving:
Net Carbs: 3.6 g Protein: 41 g
Fat: 20.5 g Calories: 380 kcal

INGREDIENTS

1 whole chicken
8 cups filtered water
3 ½ - 4 stalks celery
⅓ large red onion
1 ½ large carrot
1 zucchini, made into noodles
3 cloves garlic
2 sprigs of thyme
1-2 sprigs of rosemary
Sea salt and black pepper to taste

This is how you make the recipe

1. Clean and cut up whole chicken by separating wings, breast, backbone, legs and thighs. Remove skin from chicken breasts but keep skin on everything else.

2. Pour water into large stock pot and place cut up chicken in water.

3. Turn burner on medium-high heat. Once water reaches boil turn to medium or medium-low and simmer for about 10 minutes and then add onion, celery, garlic, salt and pepper to taste.

4. Simmer on medium-low heat for 30 minutes, then add thyme and carrots.

5. Simmer on low for another 30 minutes.

6. Once meat falls off bones skim as much of the fat that has risen to the top.

7. Once you have skimmed as much fat off the top transfer chicken with a slotted spoon to a separate bowl to debone, once deboned, return chicken meat only, to the pot and add rosemary sprigs.

8. Simmer at low heat for 10-20 minutes.

9. Serve with zucchini noodles or whatever other add-ins you like.

SAUSAGE, PEPPERS & SPINACH SOUP

Servings: 6

Nutritional Facts Per Serving:
- Net Carbs: 12.6 g
- Protein: 25.7 g
- Fat: 35.2 g
- Calories: 472.8 kcal

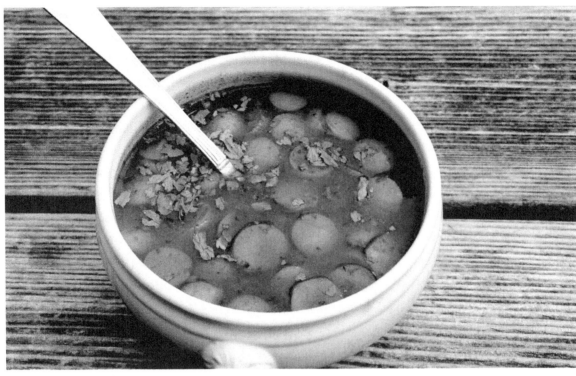

INGREDIENTS

- 2 tbsp olive oil
- 1 lb pork sausage
- 1 medium red pepper, diced
- ½ medium poblano pepper, diced
- 3 celery stalks, diced
- 1 tsp dried basil
- 1 tsp dried oregano
- 1 tsp dried rosemary
- 1½ tsp chili powder
- 1 tsp ground cumin
- ½ tsp ground cinnamon
- Sea salt and black pepper, to taste
- 6 cups sugar-free chicken stock
- 2 cups baby spinach
- 1 cup cheddar cheese, shredded

This is how you make the recipe

1. In a Dutch oven or large soup pot, heat olive oil over medium-high heat. Add sausage. Cook for approximately 5 minutes, stirring occasionally, until the sausage is no longer pink inside. Break up the sausage into small pieces with a wooden spoon as it cooks.

2. Add the peppers (red and poblano), celery, oregano, basil, rosemary, chili powder, cumin, and cinnamon into the pot. Season with salt and pepper to taste, and then stir to combine. Cook while stirring occasionally until the vegetables have softened (5-6 minutes).

3. Add chicken stock. Simmer for 20 minutes while stirring occasionally. Add spinach and cook until the spinach wilts (about 4-5 minutes).

4. Remove from heat. Serve immediately topped with cheese and, if desired, additional diced peppers.

KETO SOUP RECIPES

TOMATO BASIL SOUP

Servings: 6

Nutritional Facts Per Serving:
Net Carbs: 3 g   Protein: 3.2 g
Fat: 24.7 g   Calories: 243.7 kcal

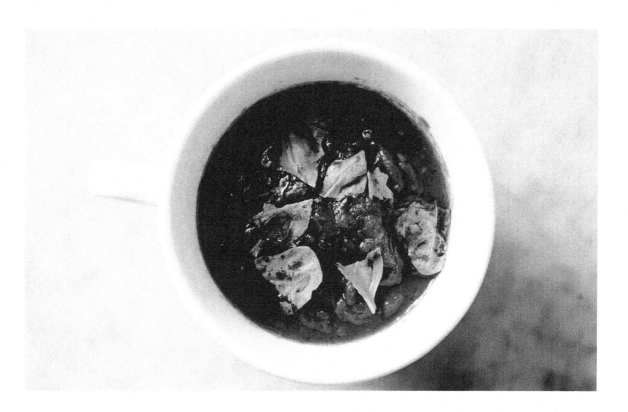

INGREDIENTS

1 can whole plum tomatoes
2 cups filtered water
1 ½ tsp coarse sea salt
½ tsp onion powder
¼ tsp garlic powder
1 tbsp butter
8 oz mascarpone cheese
2 tbsp Swerve
1 tsp apple cider vinegar
¼ tsp dried basil leaves
¼ cup prepared basil pesto, plus more for garnish (optional)

This is how you make the recipe

1. Combine the canned tomatoes, water, salt, onion powder and garlic powder in a medium saucepan.

2. Bring to a boil over medium-high heat and then simmer for 2 minutes.

3. Remove from the heat and purée with an immersion blender until smooth (or transfer to a traditional blender and blend), then return blended soup to the pan.

4. Return to the stove and add the butter and mascarpone cheese to the soup.

5. Stir over low heat until melted and creamy – about 2 minutes.

6. Remove from the heat and stir in the sweetener, apple cider vinegar, dried basil, and pesto.

7. Serve warm and enjoy!

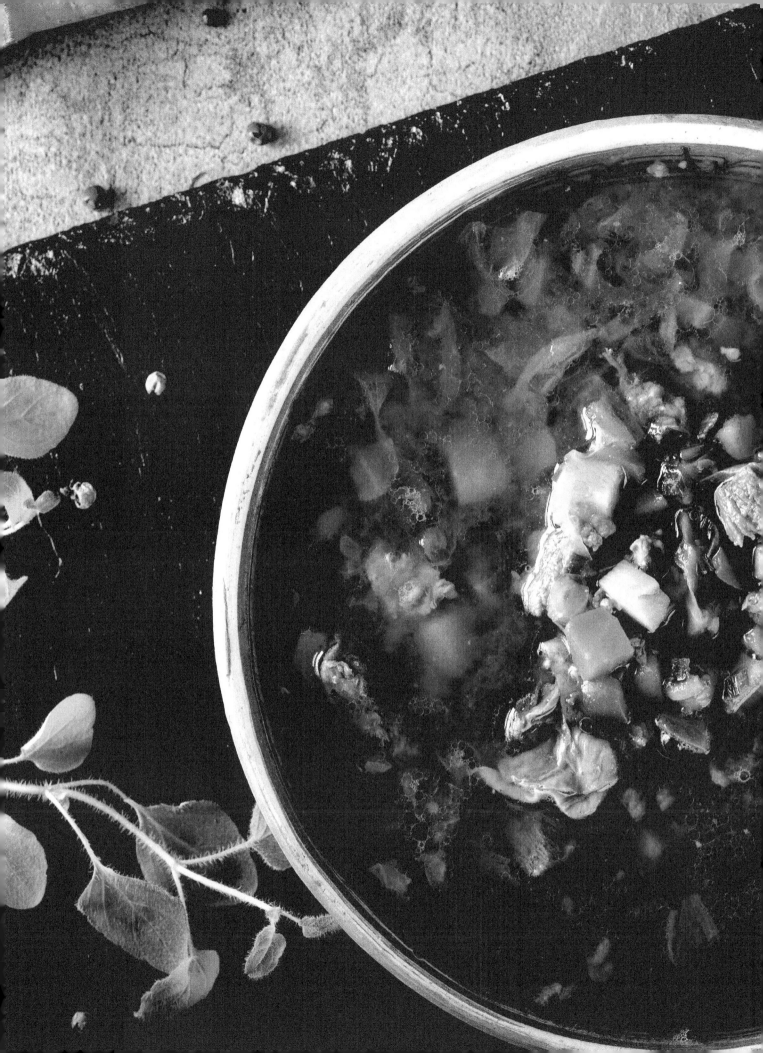

BEEF CABBAGE SOUP

Servings: 8

Nutritional Facts Per Serving:
Net Carbs: 5.6 g   Protein: 19.9 g
Fat: 17.1 g   Calories: 257.4 kcal

INGREDIENTS

2 tbsp olive oil
1 large onion, chopped
1 lb rib eye steak, cut into 1-inch pieces (trimmed of visible fat)
1 stalk celery, chopped
2 large carrots, peeled and diced
1 small green cabbage, chopped into bite-sized pieces
4 cloves garlic, minced
6 cups beef stock or broth
3 tbsp fresh chopped parsley plus more to serve
2 tsp each dried thyme and dried rosemary (or dried basil and oregano)
2 tsp onion or garlic powder
Salt and black pepper to taste

This is how you make the recipe

1. Heat oil in a large pot over medium-heat, add the beef and sear on all sides until browned all over (they don't need to be cooked through). Then add the onions and cook until transparent (about 3-4 minutes).

2. Add the celery and carrots to the pan, mixing through the flavors in the pot. Cook while mixing occasionally for about 3-4 minutes, then add the cabbage and cook for a further 5 minutes until beginning to soften; add in the garlic, and cook until fragrant (about 1 minute), mixing all ingredients through.

3. Add the stock (or broth), parsley, dried herbs, and onion or garlic powder; mixing well. Bring to a simmer; reduce heat to medium-low and cover, with a lid.

4. Allow to simmer for 10-15 minutes, or until the cabbage and carrots are soft. Season with salt and pepper, and add in a little extra dried herbs, if needed.

5. Serve warm with a sprinkle of fresh parsley (if desired).

KETO SOUP RECIPES

CREAMY PUMPKIN & SAUSAGE CHOWDER

Servings: 8

Nutritional Facts Per Serving:
Net Carbs: 5.3 g   Protein: 13.1 g
Fat: 28.8 g   Calories: 333.1 kcal

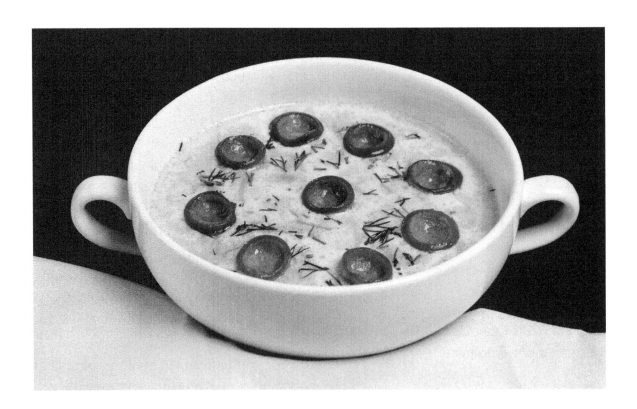

INGREDIENTS

1 lb pork sausage roll
1 ¼ cup pumpkin purée
3 cups water
1 tsp sea salt
¼ tsp ground nutmeg
¼ tsp ground black pepper
1 tsp garlic powder
1 tsp onion powder
3 cups cauliflower rice
1 tbsp minced fresh sage
8 oz mascarpone cheese

This is how you make the recipe

1. Brown the sausage in a large saucepan, stirring to break it up into small pieces.

2. Add the chicken broth, pumpkin purée, water, salt, nutmeg, pepper, garlic, onion, and cauliflower. Simmer 20 minutes.

3. Add the mascarpone cheese and sage. Cook over medium-low heat, stirring occasionally, for five minutes or until the cheese has melted into the broth and is creamy and smooth. Do not boil.

4. Serve and enjoy!

CHIPOTLE AVOCADO SOUP

Servings: 4

Nutritional Facts Per Serving:
Net Carbs: 2.3 g   Protein: 2.9 g
Fat: 29.2 g   Calories: 288 kcal

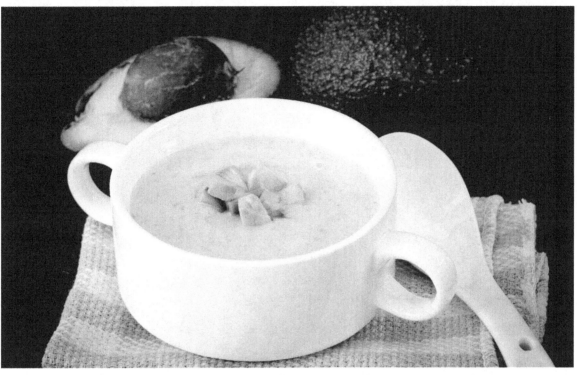

INGREDIENTS

2 large ripe avocados
3 cups chicken stock or vegetable broth
1 cup full-fat sour cream
½-1 tsp (or to taste) chipotle
Sea salt to taste

This is how you make the recipe

1. Halve the avocados. Remove the pits and discard them. Place the flesh into a blender.

2. Blend the avocados until smooth. Add some stock to help the blending process, if necessary.

3. In a large saucepan, bring the rest of the stock to a boil, then remove from the heat.

4. Add the avocado mash, sour cream, and chipotle. Mix well with a spoon until smooth. If there are lumps, use an immersion blender or regular blender to blend the soup until very smooth.

5. Heat again until hot, but don't let it boil (this is very important! If the mixture boils, it might separate).

6. Season with salt if desired.

7. Divide the soup into soup bowls.

8. Serve with lemon or lime wedges and chopped fresh herbs (like parsley or cilantro) if desired.

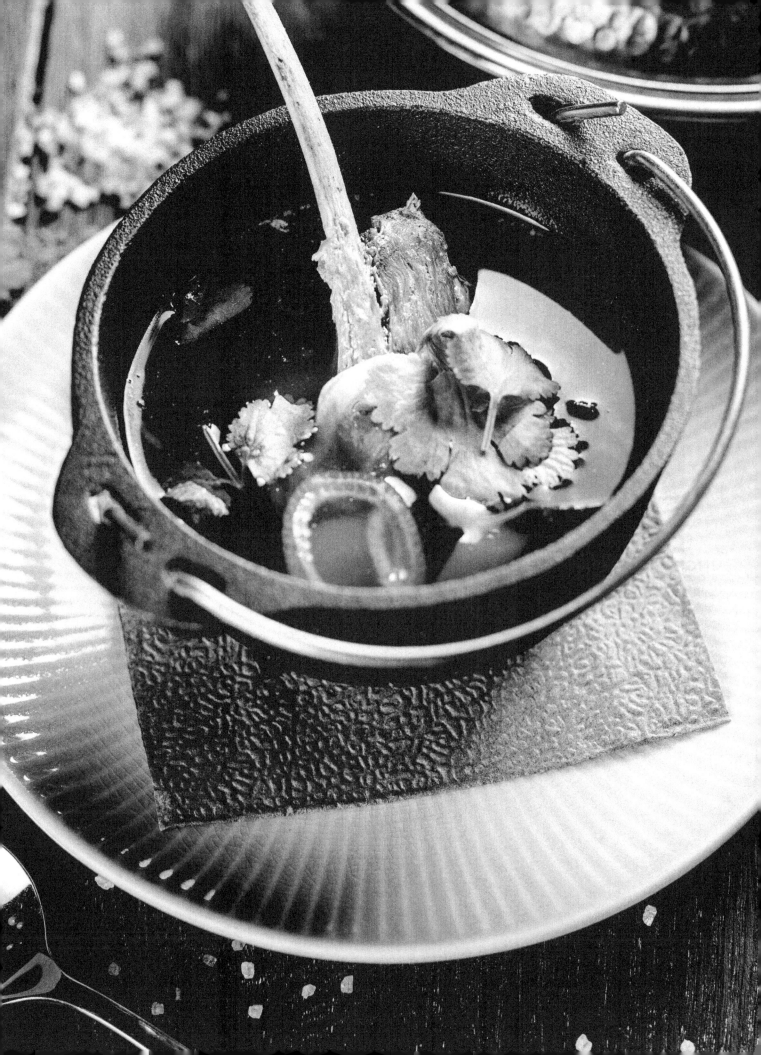

LAMB & HERB BONE BROTH

Servings: 4

Nutritional Facts Per Serving:
Net Carbs: 4.8 g Protein: 28.8 g
Fat: 27.5 g Calories: 394.3 kcal

INGREDIENTS

1 lb lamb bones
1 tbsp olive oil
1 small onion large, diced
3 medium carrots, cut into chunks
3 sticks celery, roughly chopped
3 cloves garlic
3 sprigs rosemary
5 sprigs thyme
1-3 gallons water
Sea salt (optional)

This is how you make the recipe

1. Preheat oven to 390°F.
2. Place lamb bones into a roasting pan and cook for 30-40 minutes, until well browned.
3. In a large stock pot, add the oil and place over medium heat.
4. Add the onion, carrot, celery, garlic, thyme and rosemary and sauté for 5 minutes.
5. Add the lamb bones and scrape any fat or juices from the roasting pan into the pot.
6. Add 1 gallon of water and allow to come to a simmer before reducing the heat to low.
7. Simmer for 8-24 hours uncovered, adding more water when the level drops. The amount of water you need will depend on how long you wish to cook the broth for.
8. After the broth is cooked for your desired length of time, strain the broth through a fine mesh strainer.
9. Enjoy hot or chill and use as desired.

KETO SOUP RECIPES

CHICKEN POBLANO SOUP

Servings: 8

Nutritional Facts Per Serving:
Net Carbs: 7.6 g   Protein: 29.6 g
Fat: 5.9 g   Calories: 218.5 kcal

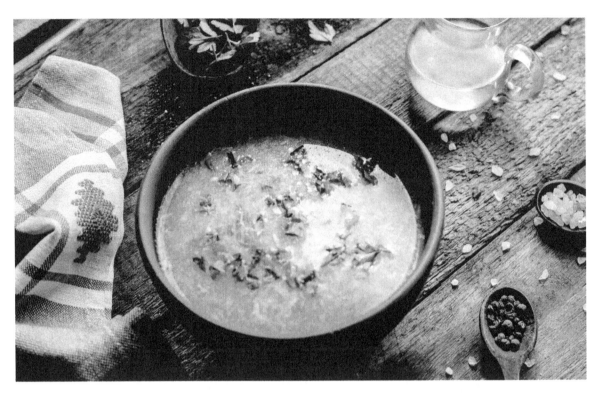

INGREDIENTS

1 cup onion diced
3 poblano peppers, chopped
5 cloves garlic
1 cup cauliflower, diced
1 ½ lb chicken breast, large chunks
¼ cup cilantro, chopped
1 tsp ground coriander
1 tsp ground cumin
1-2 tsp sea salt
2 ½ cups water
2 oz cream cheese

This is how you make the recipe

1. Put everything except the cream cheese into your Instant pot, and cook at high pressure for 15 minutes. Allow it to release pressure naturally for ten minutes, and the release all remaining pressure.

2. Remove chicken with tongs and using an immersion blender, roughly purée the soup and vegetables.

3. Turn your pot onto sauté, and when the broth is hot and bubbling, put in the cream cheese cut into chunks. Use a whisk to blend in the cream cheese if needed.

4. Shred the chicken and put back into the pot, until heated through.

5. You can also purée the vegetables and chicken together, to get a thicker, more robust soup.

6. Serve and enjoy!

EASY CHICKEN SOUP

Servings: 8

Nutritional Facts Per Serving:
Net Carbs: 15.3 g Protein: 25.3 g
Fat: 8.3 g Calories: 253.3 kcal

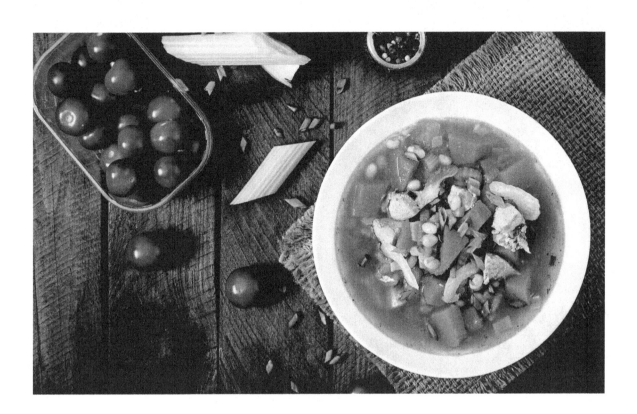

INGREDIENTS

10 cups bone broth or chicken stock
½ tsp garlic powder
½ tsp dried oregano
1 cup thinly-sliced celery
1 ½ cups diced butternut squash
2 cups jicama, peeled and chopped small
4 cups cooked, shredded or chopped chicken
¼ cup chopped fresh parsley
1 tbsp apple cider vinegar
Sea salt and pepper to taste

This is how you make the recipe

1. Combine the broth, garlic powder, dried oregano, celery, butternut squash and jicama in a large pot.

2. Bring to a boil, then lower heat and simmer (uncovered) for 30 minutes, or until veggies are fork tender.

3. Add the chicken and cook for another 5 minutes, or until heated through (don't cook the chicken too long or it will get tough.)

4. Remove from the heat and add the parsley and apple cider vinegar.

5. Season with sea salt and pepper to taste before serving.

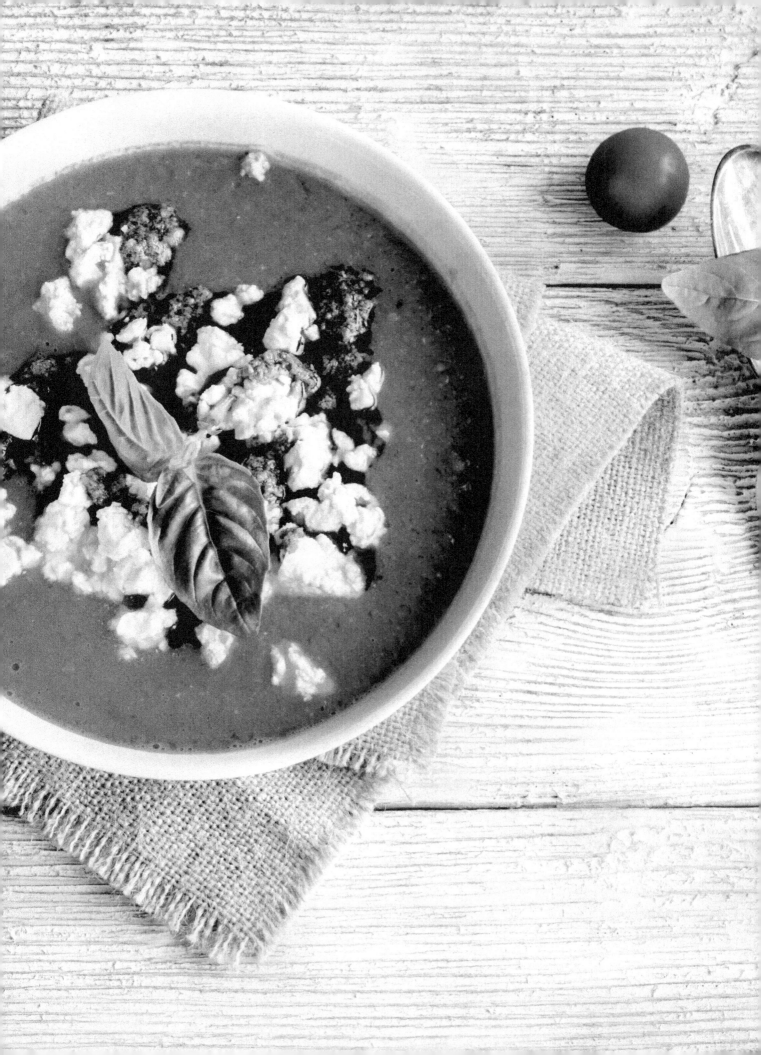

TOMATO FETA SOUP

Servings: 6

Nutritional Facts Per Serving:
Net Carbs: 8 g
Protein: 4 g
Fat: 13 g
Calories: 170 kcal

INGREDIENTS

2 tbsp olive oil or butter
¼ cup onion, chopped
2 cloves garlic
½ tsp salt
⅛ tsp black pepper
1 tsp pesto sauce (optional)
½ tsp dried oregano
1 tsp dried basil
1 tbsp tomato paste (optional)
10 tomatoes, skinned, seeded and chopped
1 tsp Swerve or sweetener of choice (optional)
3 cups water
⅓ cup heavy cream
⅔ cup feta cheese, crumbled

This is how you make the recipe

1. Heat olive oil (butter) over medium heat in a large pot (Dutch Oven). Add the onion and cook for 2 minutes, stirring frequently. Add the garlic and cook for 1 minute. Add tomatoes, salt, pepper, pesto (optional), oregano, basil, tomato paste and water. Bring to a boil, then reduce to a simmer. Add sweetener.

2. Cook on medium heat for 20 minutes, until the tomatoes are tender. Using an immersion blender, blend until smooth. Add the cream and feta cheese. Cook for 1 more minute.

3. Add more salt if needed. Serve and enjoy!

KETO SOUP RECIPES

SHIRATAKI PHO

Servings: 6

Nutritional Facts Per Serving:
Net Carbs: 7 g Protein: 60.5 g
Fat: 40.7 g Calories: 642 kcal

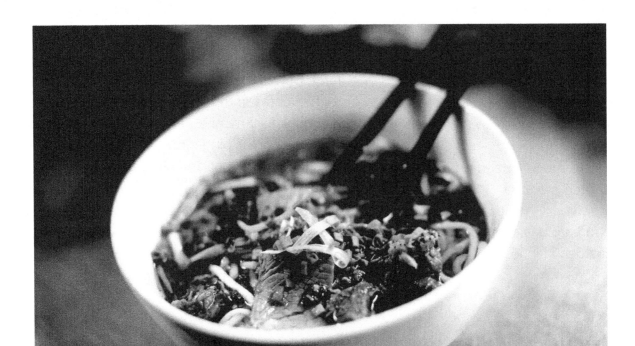

INGREDIENTS

1 gallon filtered water
2 lb beef short ribs
1 lb flank steak cut into thin strips
1 tbsp chicken bouillon cube
1 ½ tsp sea salt
1 lb shirataki noodles
2 large red onions
Thai basil, lime juice, soy sauce and chili paste for garnish (optional)

This is how you make the recipe

1. To a large pot, add 1 gallon of water and bring to a boil. Lower the heat to medium-low and add your ribs, salt and bouillon cube. Cover and let simmer.

2. Cut your onions in half, remove the skin and place on a baking sheet. Using a blow torch, roast the exposed part of your onions until it gets black. If you don't have a blow torch, use the broil function of your oven to roast your onions.

3. Add your onions to the pot and let simmer for 2 hours or until your ribs are very tender. The meat should come right off the bone.

4. Assembly: In a large bowl, place your shirataki noodles, 4-5 thin slices of steak, some short-rib meat and a handful of Thai basil. Make sure that your broth if very hot, so that it will cook your steak perfectly to medium rare.

5. Serve and enjoy!

PORK & TOMATO SOUP

Servings: 8

Nutritional Facts Per Serving:
Net Carbs: 3 g Protein: 21 g
Fat: 22 g Calories: 326 kcal

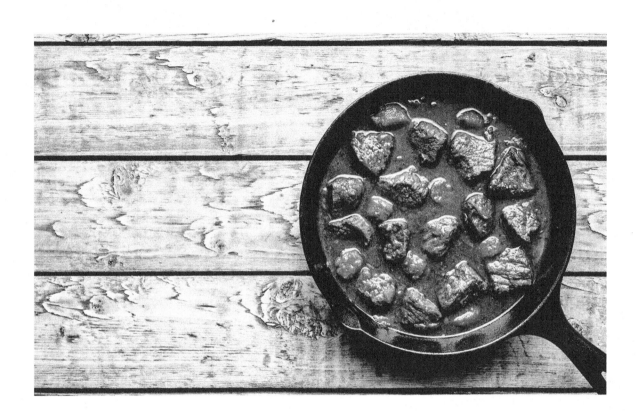

INGREDIENTS

2 lb boneless country pork ribs, cut into 1-inch pieces
1 tbsp olive oil
1 tbsp chopped garlic
½ cup chopped onion
½ cup dry white wine
1 cup chicken stock
2 cups fresh tomatoes, chopped
1 cup water
2 tbsp fresh oregano, chopped
2 cups finely chopped cauliflower
Sea salt and black pepper to taste

This is how you make the recipe

1. Heat the olive oil in a heavy saucepan. Season the pork (or other meat) generously with salt and pepper.

2. Brown the meat on all sides for several minutes or until golden.

3. Add the garlic and onions and cook for 2 minutes.

4. Add the white wine, chicken stock, fresh tomatoes and water and bring to a boil.

5. Pour into a slow cooker and cook on high for 4 hours or until the meat is tender and falling apart.

6. In the last 15-20 minutes of cooking, stir in the cauliflower and fresh oregano. Serve hot and enjoy!

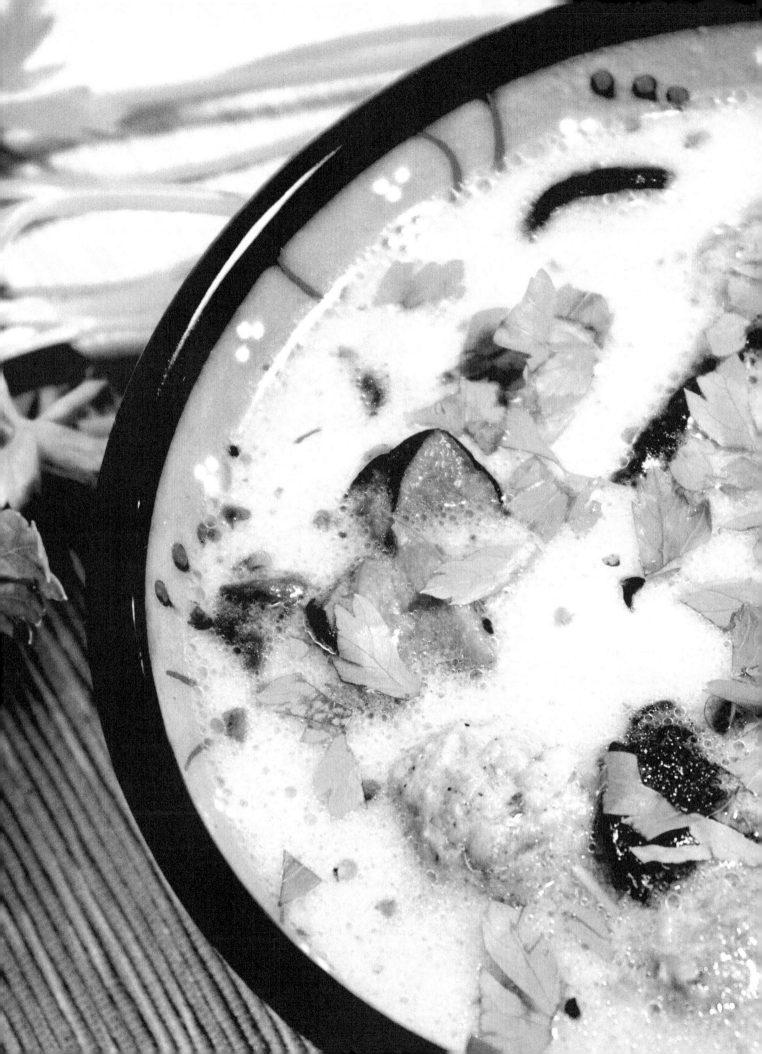

ONE-POT CREAMY MEATBALL SOUP

Servings: 14

Nutritional Facts Per Serving:
Net Carbs: 7 g Protein: 19.5 g
Fat: 31 g Calories: 384 kcal

INGREDIENTS

For the Meatballs:
1 lb ground pork
1 lb ground Italian sausage, mild or spicy, depending on your preference
½ cup very finely minced onion
1 tbsp minced garlic
1 stalk celery, finely minced
1 egg

For the Soup:
2 lb meatballs (above recipe)
1 large onion, diced
¼ cup diced garlic
8 oz cremini mushrooms, cleaned and sliced into thin rounds
Sea salt and black pepper, to taste
2 large carrots, peeled, then sliced into thin rounds
3 large stalks celery, sliced into thin half-rounds
1 ½ cups beef stock
1 tbsp Italian herb seasoning blend
2 cups heavy whipping cream
1 cup grated parmesan cheese

This is how you make the recipe

1. For the meatballs: Combine meatball ingredients in a large bowl and mix well.
2. Roll into golfball sized balls.
3. Let chill 1 hour in refrigerator to set.
4. For the soup: Add olive oil to pan or Dutch oven, and heat on medium-high until shimmery.
5. Add meatballs and brown on all sides, about 3-5 minutes per side.
6. When meatballs are lightly browned on all sides, remove from pan and set aside.
7. Add onions, garlic, carrots, mushrooms, and celery to pot or Dutch oven.
8. Brown vegetables until soft, another 5-8 minutes.
9. Add stock, herbs, and meatballs to pot and increase heat to high.
10. Let stock reduce down by half.
11. Turn heat off and slowly add in cream, whisking as it is added.
12. Whisk vigorously to incorporate into soup.
13. Return heat to medium and whisk in parmesan cheese.
14. Let come to a rolling boil and thicken, another 2-4 minutes.
15. When soup is thickened, serve.

KETO SOUP RECIPES

EASY TACO SOUP

Servings: 8

Nutritional Facts Per Serving:
Net Carbs: 7.4 g   Protein: 34.8 g
Fat: 29.9 g   Calories: 445.1 kcal

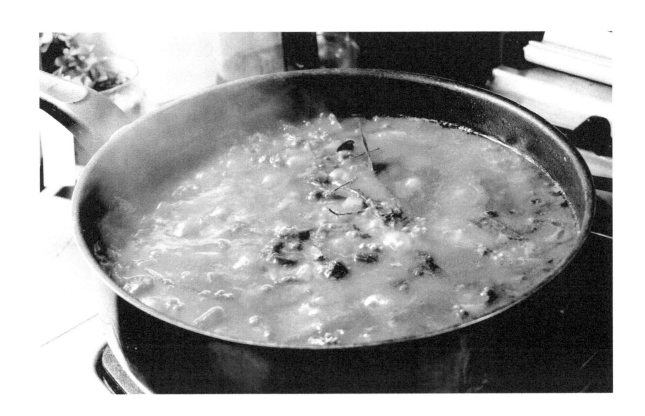

INGREDIENTS

2 lb ground beef
2 cloves garlic, minced
½ cup onion, diced
2 tbsp homemade taco seasoning
½ tsp ancho chili powder
2 (10 oz) cans Ro-tel with green peppers
8 oz block cream cheese
½ cup fresh cilantro, chopped
4 cups beef broth

This is how you make the recipe

1. In a skillet on the stove, crumble and cook ground beef, diced onion, and garlic.

2. Transfer ground beef mixture to slow cooker. Add seasonings and remaining ingredients.

3. Close lid and cook on low for 4 hours, or 2 hours on high.

4. Serve with your choice of toppings and enjoy!

KETO SOUP RECIPES

CREAMY BROCCOLI & CHEDDAR SOUP

Servings: 6

Nutritional Facts Per Serving:
Net Carbs: 5.8 g Protein: 13.3 g
Fat: 28.3 g Calories: 335.2 kcal

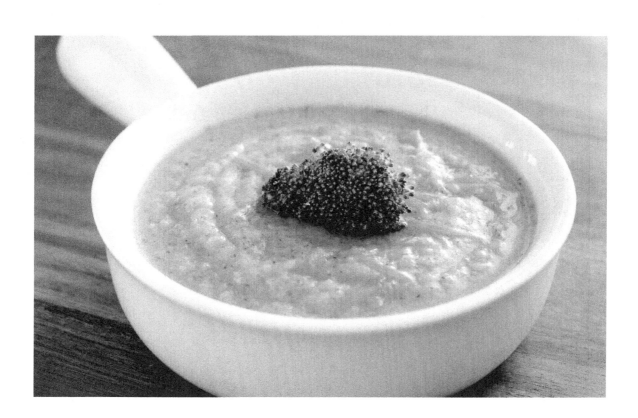

INGREDIENTS

4 cups broccoli florets
2 cups beef broth
1 cup sharp cheddar cheese, shredded
½ tsp garlic powder
½ tsp onion powder
½ tsp mustard powder
⅛ tsp nutmeg
½ tsp sea salt or to taste
¼ tsp ground black pepper
½ cup heavy whipping cream
¼ cup butter

This is how you make the recipe

1. Cook the broccoli florets by steaming them on the stove.

2. Combine the broccoli and other ingredients in a blender and blend until mostly smooth.

3. Add to a pot and simmer on the stove for about 10 minutes.

4. Serve hot and enjoy!

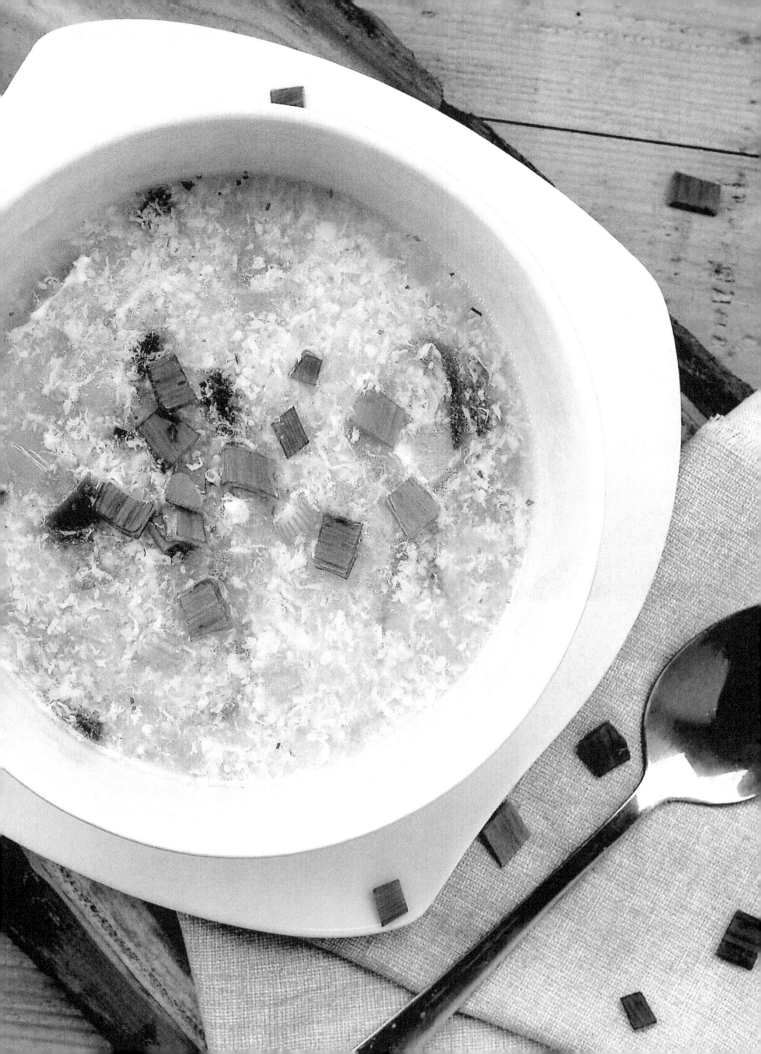

ANTI-INFLAMMATORY EGG-DROP SOUP

Servings: 6

Nutritional Facts Per Serving:
Net Carbs: 18.7 g Protein: 16.2 g
Fat: 21 g Calories: 337.2 kcal

INGREDIENTS

8 cups chicken stock, vegetable stock or bone broth
1 tbsp freshly grated turmeric or 1 tsp ground turmeric
1 tbsp freshly grated ginger or 1 tsp ground ginger
2 cloves garlic, minced
1 small chili pepper, sliced
2 tbsp coconut aminos
2 cups sliced brown mushrooms
4 cups chopped Swiss chard or spinach
4 large eggs
2 medium spring onions, sliced
2 tbsp freshly chopped cilantro
Sea salt and black pepper to taste
6 tbsp olive oil

This is how you make the recipe

1. Grate the turmeric and ginger root, slice the chili pepper and mince the garlic cloves.

2. Pour the chicken stock (or vegetable stock) in a large pot and heat over a medium heat, until it starts to simmer. Slice the mushrooms, chard stalks and chard leaves. Place the turmeric, ginger, garlic, chili pepper, mushrooms, chard stalks and coconut aminos into the pot and simmer for about 5 minutes

3. Then add the sliced chard leaves and cook for another minute. In a bowl, whisk the eggs and slowly pour them into the simmering soup.

4. Keep stirring until the egg is cooked and take off the heat. Chop the cilantro and slice the spring onions. Add them to the pot. Season with salt and pepper to taste.

5. Pour into a serving bowl and drizzle with olive oil (a tbsp per serving). Enjoy!

KETO SOUP RECIPES

HAM & CABBAGE SOUP

Servings: 6-8

Nutritional Facts Per Serving:
Net Carbs: 15.2 g   Protein: 14.5 g
Fat: 4.1 g   Calories: 163.5 kcal

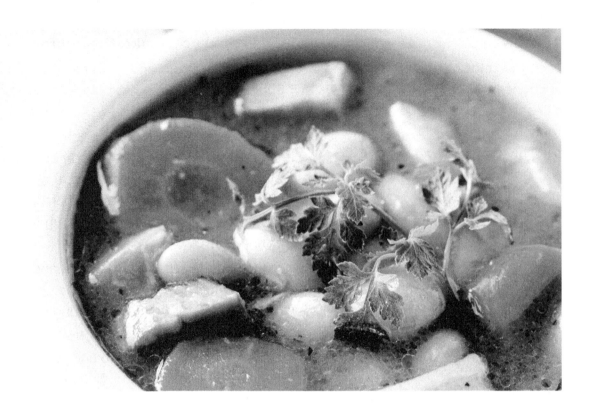

INGREDIENTS

1 head cabbage, chopped
1 onion, finely chopped
1 red bell pepper, finely chopped
2 small carrots, cut in small rounds or chopped
2 cups diced lean ham
2 bay leaves
1 tsp Spike Seasoning
1 tsp granulated garlic
1 tbsp dried parsley
1 tsp sea salt
Black pepper to taste
6 cups chicken stock
2 packets Goya Ham Flavor Concentrate or other ham flavor base
Parmesan cheese for serving

This is how you make the recipe

1. Chop cabbage, onion, red bell pepper, ham, and carrots.

2. Put cabbage, onion, and red bell pepper in the bottom of the Instant pot. Add the chopped ham, carrots, and bay leaves, and sprinkle the Spike Seasoning, granulated garlic, dried parsley, sea salt, and black pepper over the top.

3. Mix the Goya Ham Flavor Concentrate or other ham flavor base into the chicken stock and pour the liquid over the ingredients in the Instant pot.

4. Lock the lid, set to manual, high pressure, and cook for 15 minutes.

5. Let pressure release manually for 10-15 minutes, then release manually. Discard bay leaves.

6. Serve hot, with freshly grated parmesan to add at the table if desired.

CREAMY VEGETABLE SOUP

Servings: 8

Nutritional Facts Per Serving:
Net Carbs: 14.3 g Protein: 10.1 g
Fat: 23.5 g Calories: 311.9 kcal

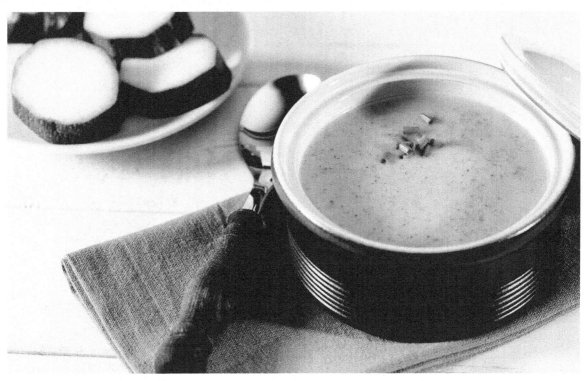

INGREDIENTS

1 ½ lb cauliflower
1 lb zucchini
1 clove garlic
1 small brown onion
2 celery stalks
2 tbsp ghee or butter
2 cups chicken broth or vegetable stock
2 cups filtered water
1 tsp fresh thyme, plus extra for garnish
½ tsp onion powder
Sea salt and black pepper to taste
1 cup cream
4 tbsp olive oil

This is how you make the recipe

1. Wash the vegetables. Remove the green parts of the cauliflower. Peel the onion and garlic.

2. Heat the ghee over medium to high heat in a large saucepan. Chop the onion and garlic finely and sauté until translucent.

3. Add chopped cauliflower, zucchini, celery and seasonings.

4. Add broth and water and bring to the boil. Place a lid on the saucepan and reduce to a simmer. Cook until vegetables are soft, for about 15 minutes.

5. Remove from heat and use an immersion mixer to purée until smooth. Add cream and return to heat until heated through.

6. Serve with a drizzle of olive oil (about ½ tbsp per serving) and a sprig of thyme.

7. Serve ad enjoy!

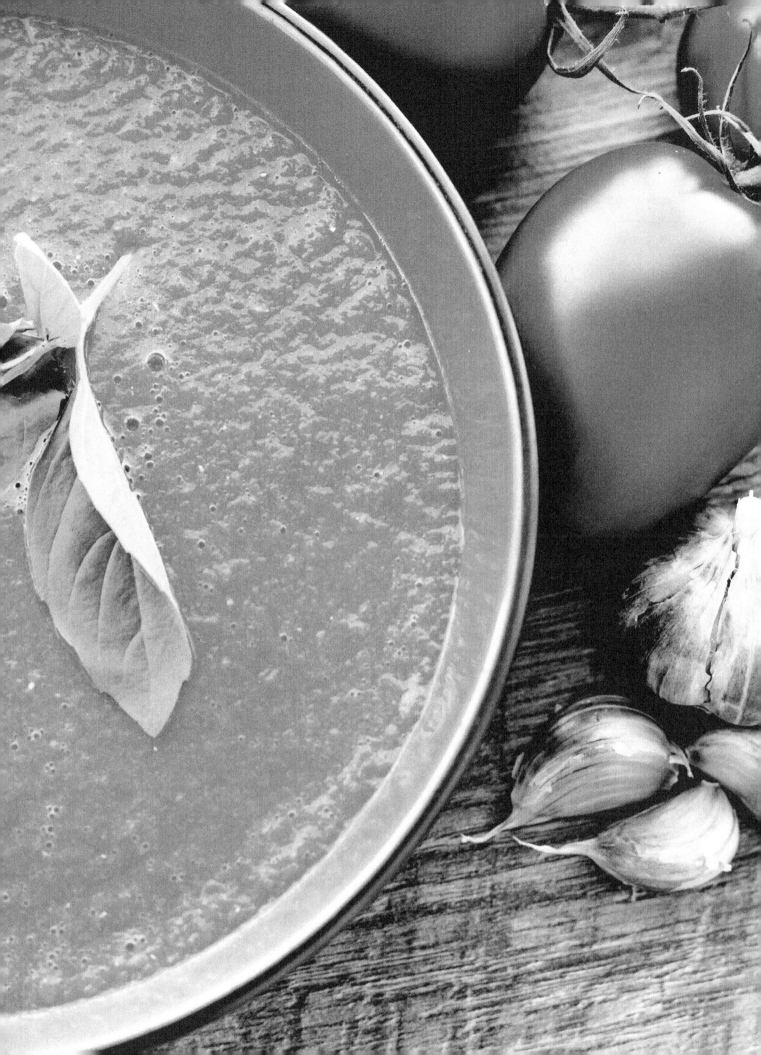

ROASTED TOMATO & GARLIC SOUP

Servings: 4

Nutritional Facts Per Serving:
Net Carbs: 5.4 g Protein: 3 g
Fat: 14.5 g Calories: 163.8 kcal

INGREDIENTS

1 lb fresh tomatoes, cored
4 cloves garlic, peeled
2 tbsp olive oil
½ tsp sea salt
¼ tsp ground black pepper
4 cups chicken broth
2 tbsp olive oil
⅛th tsp ground nutmeg
¼ tsp anchovy paste
2 bay leaves
1 tsp apple cider vinegar
Sea salt and black pepper to taste

This is how you make the recipe

1. Preheat the oven to 400°F.
2. Place the cored tomatoes and peeled garlic on a cookie sheet.
3. Drizzle with 2 tbsp of olive oil, salt and pepper.
4. Roast for 30 minutes.
5. Remove and transfer vegetables and any pan juices to a blender.
6. Add 2 cups of chicken stock and blend until smooth.
7. Pour through a strainer (to remove seeds and skin pieces) into a large saucepan.
8. Add the remaining 2 cups of chicken stock, 2 tbsp olive oil, nutmeg, anchovy paste and bay leaves.
9. Simmer over medium heat for 10 minutes.
10. Remove the bay leaves.
11. Add apple cider vinegar.
12. Stir and taste, season with additional salt and pepper as desired.

CREAMY REUBEN SOUP

Servings: 14

Nutritional Facts Per Serving:
Net Carbs: 3.2 g   Protein: 13.3 g
Fat: 25 g   Calories: 285.5 kcal

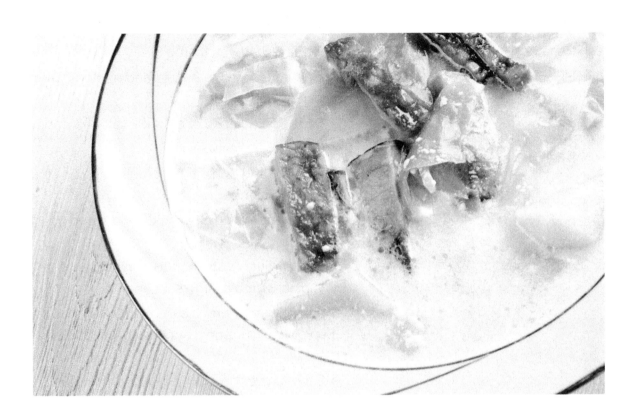

INGREDIENTS

1 medium onion, diced
2 ribs celery, diced
2 large cloves garlic, minced
3 tbsp butter
1 lb corned beef, chopped
4 cups beef stock
1 cup sauerkraut
1 tsp sea salt
1 tsp caraway seeds
¾ tsp black pepper
2 cups heavy cream
1 ½ cup Swiss cheese, shredded

This is how you make the recipe

1. Heat slow cooker on high setting.

2. To a large sauté pan, over medium-low heat, add onion, celery, garlic and butter. Sauté until soft and translucent. Transfer to slow cooker.

3. To the slow cooker, add corned beef, beef stock, sauerkraut, sea salt, caraway seed and black pepper. Cover and cook on high for 4 ½ hours.

4. Add heavy cream and Swiss cheese and cook 1 additional hour.

5. Serve and enjoy!

CHICKEN RAMEN

Servings: 4

Nutritional Facts Per Serving:
Net Carbs: 9.8 g Protein: 90.5 g
Fat: 49.5 g Calories: 871 kcal

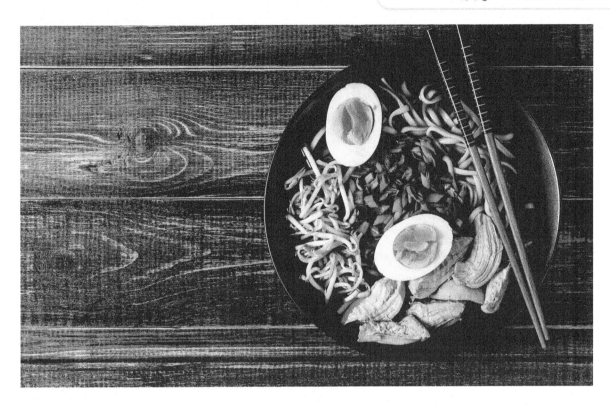

INGREDIENTS

1 small chicken
12 cups filter water
2 chicken broth cubes
4 large eggs
2 tbsp sea salt
2 packs shirataki noodles
6 green onions chopped
4 tbsp gluten-free soy sauce

This is how you make the recipe

1. In a large pot, bring your water to a boil and add your chicken to it. Lower the heat to medium-low, add your chicken stock cubes and salt. Cover and cook for 1 hour and 15 minutes.

2. Remove your chicken from the pot, leave your broth uncovered and let it simmer for another 45 minutes on low heat. Once your broth is ready, pass through a strainer to get rid of any impurities.

3. Once your chicken has cooled down, strip off all its meat from bones and place it in a bowl.

4. In a medium pot, bring 4 cups of water to a boil and carefully place your 4 eggs in there. Cook for exactly 6 minutes for perfectly runny egg yolks.

5. For each bowl, place half a pack of shirataki noodles, 1 tbsp of soy sauce, as much chicken as you like, 1 soft boiled egg cut in half of course and a handful of chopped green onions.

6. Serve and enjoy!

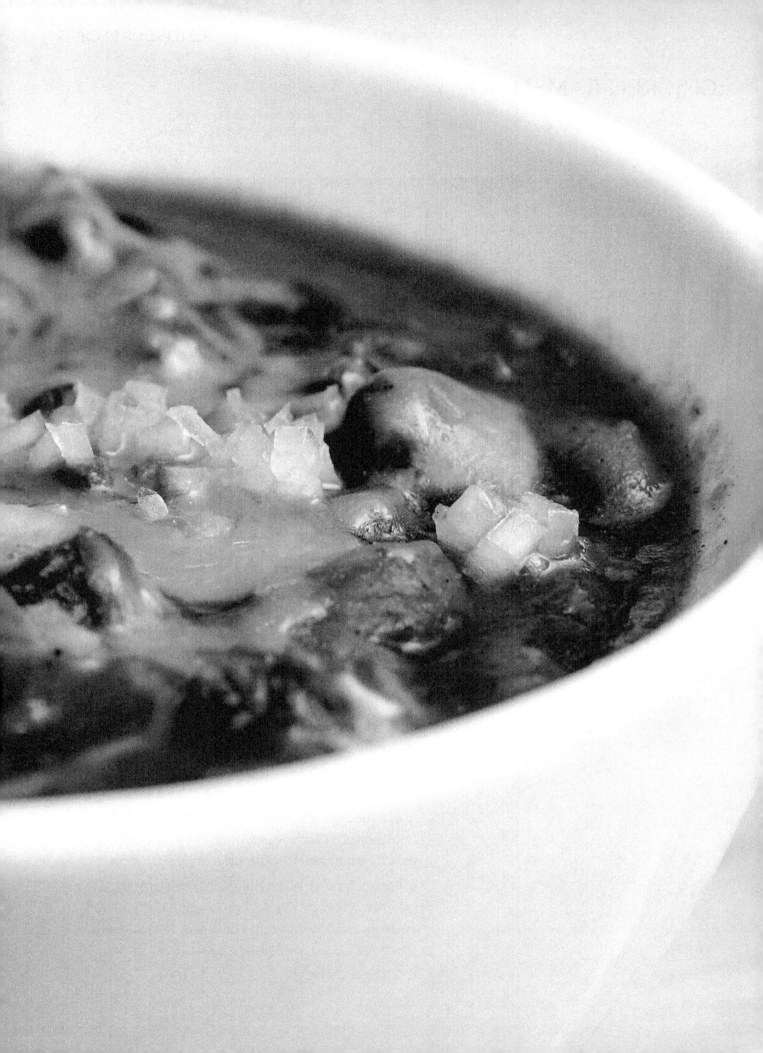

BACON CHEESEBURGER SOUP

Servings: 12

Nutritional Facts Per Serving:
Net Carbs: 3 g Protein: 13 g
Fat: 11 g Calories: 306 kcal

INGREDIENTS

4 cups beef stock
1 medium tomato, diced
⅓ cup chopped dill pickles
2 tbsp Dijon Mustard
2 tbsp Worcestershire sauce
2 tbsp chopped fresh flat-leaf parsley
1 tsp sea salt, more to taste
½ tsp black pepper
1 ½ lb ground beef
1 small onion, diced
4 cloves garlic, minced
1 ½ cups shredded sharp cheddar cheese
1 cup heavy cream
8 slices bacon, cooked crisp and crumbled

This is how you make the recipe

1. Slow cooker: Heat the slow cooker on low setting.

2. To the slow cooker, add the beef stock, tomato, pickles, Dijon, Worcestershire sauce, parsley, sea salt, and black pepper.

3. In a large skillet, over medium-high heat, cook the ground beef, onions, and garlic until the ground beef is browned and cooked all the way through. Drain the excess grease and add to the slow cooker. Cover and cook for 6 hours.

4. Mix in cheddar cheese and heavy cream and and cook 1 additional hour.

5. Add bacon just before serving.

6. Stovetop: Heat a large Dutch oven or stock pot over medium heat. Add the ground beef, onions, and garlic, and cook until the ground beef is browned and cooked through.

7. Add the beef stock, tomato, pickles, Dijon, Worcestershire sauce, parsley, sea salt, and black pepper. Bring to a boil, and then reduce the heat to medium-low and simmer for 30 minutes.

8. Mix in the cheddar cheese and heavy cream, reduce the heat to low, cover and stirring occasionally, simmer for 30 minutes.

9. Add bacon just before serving.

KETO SOUP RECIPES

EGG-DROP SOUP

Servings: 4

Nutritional Facts Per Serving:
Net Carbs: 1.9 g   Protein: 4.75 g
Fat: 2.75 g   Calories: 52 kcal

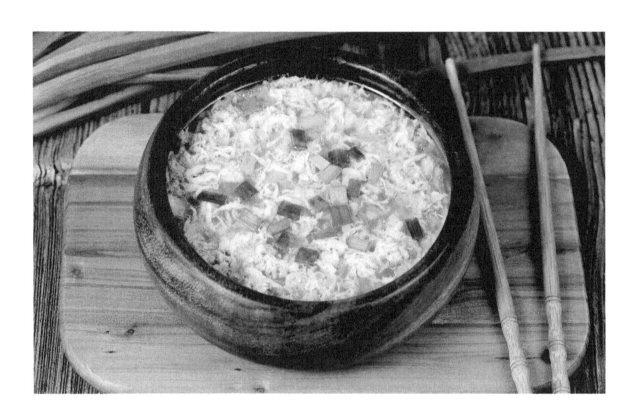

INGREDIENTS

4 cups chicken broth
1 tsp ground ginger
1 tbsp soy sauce
2 eggs, beaten
¼ cup green onions, chopped
Sea salt and black pepper

This is how you make the recipe

1. Add chicken broth, ground ginger and soy sauce to a saucepan; bring to a simmer.

2. Slowly stream in beaten eggs while stirring the soup in one direction.

3. Add green onions. Salt and pepper to taste.

4. For a spiced up version, add a bit of sriracha hot sauce or ground red pepper to taste.

5. Serve and enjoy!

MEATBALL ZOODLE SOUP

Servings: 12

Nutritional Facts Per Serving:
Net Carbs: 3.8 g   Protein: 19.2 g
Fat: 11.6 g   Calories: 201.8 kcal

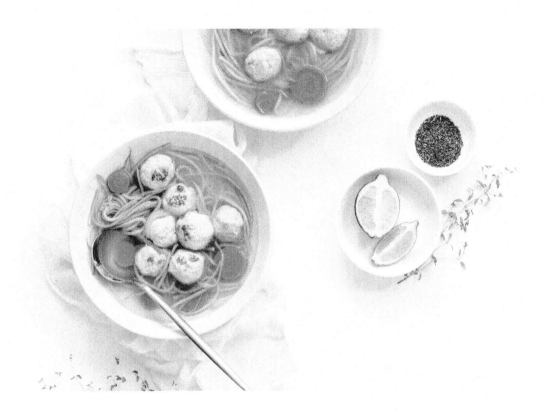

INGREDIENTS

4 cups beef stock
1 medium zucchini, spiraled
2 ribs celery, chopped
1 small onion, diced
1 carrot, chopped
1 medium tomato, diced
1 ½ tsp garlic salt
1 ½ lb ground beef
½ cup parmesan cheese, shredded
6 cloves garlic, minced
1 large egg
4 tbsp fresh parsley, chopped
1 ½ tsp sea salt
1 ½ tsp onion powder
1 tsp Italian seasoning
1 tsp dried oregano
½ tsp black pepper

This is how you make the recipe

1. Heat slow cooker on low setting.

2. To the slow cooker, add beef stock, zucchini, celery, onion, carrot, tomato, and garlic salt. Cover.

3. In a large mixing bowl, combine ground beef, parmesan, garlic, egg, parsley, sea salt, onion powder, oregano, Italian seasoning, and pepper. Mix until all ingredients are well incorporated. Form into approximately 30 meatballs.

4. Heat olive oil in a large skillet over medium-high heat. Once the pan is hot, add meatballs and brown on all sides. No need to worry about cooking them all the way through as they will be going into the slow cooker. Add meatballs to slow cooker, cover and cook for 6 hours.

5. Serve and enjoy!

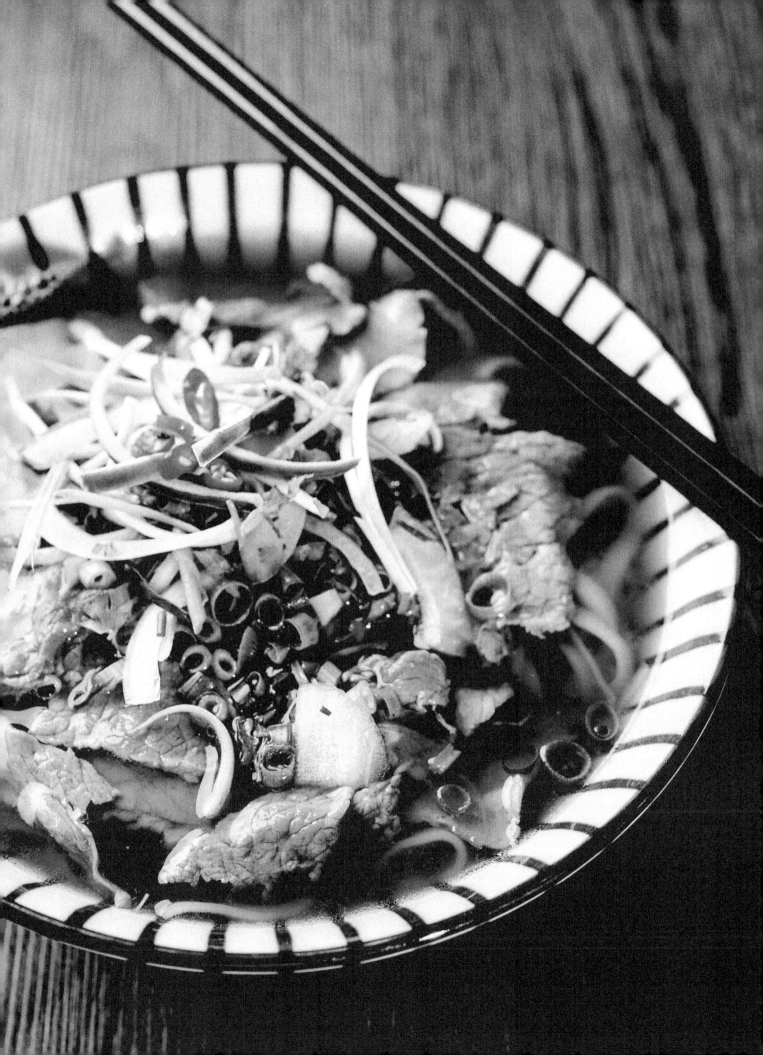

ASIAN BEEF NOODLE SOUP

Servings: 4

Nutritional Facts Per Serving:
Net Carbs: 19.1 g Protein: 43.8 g
Fat: 15.3 g Calories: 396 kcal

INGREDIENTS

½ tsp sesame oil
1 tsp black bean paste
1 clove garlic, minced
2-inch chunk of ginger, peeled and roughly chopped
1 piece of lime peel, about 1-inch by 2-inches long
2 tbsp sugar free fish sauce
6 cups beef stock or broth
1-inch piece of habanero, no seeds
1 tsp Swerve
1 tbsp lime juice
Sea salt and black pepper to taste
2 packs zero carb shirataki noodles
4 cups shredded cabbage
1 lb lean beef, thinly-sliced
½ cup shiitake mushrooms, thinly-sliced
½ cup fresh cilantro, roughly chopped
½ cup scallions, thinly-sliced
2 tbsp fresh hot chili peppers, thinly-sliced
Fresh lime for garnish

This is how you make the recipe

1. For the broth: Heat sesame oil in a medium soup pot. Add the bean paste, garlic, ginger, and lime peel and sauté for 1 minute or until fragrant.

2. Add the fish sauce, beef stock, and habanero (if using.)

3. Simmer for at least 30 minutes, preferably longer for the best flavor to develop.

4. Strain out the bits so only the broth remains. Add the Swerve and lime juice to the broth. Taste and adjust to your preference for sweet and salty.

5. To make the soup: Divide the noodles, cabbage, beef, mushrooms, cilantro, scallions and chili pepper slices between four large soup bowls.

6. Bring the broth to a boil and pour (approximately 1 ½ cups per bowl) over the soup ingredients. Let sit for 5 minutes before eating.

7. Alternate soup method: Add the noodles, cabbage and mushrooms to the boiling broth and simmer for 5-10 minutes.

8. Add the beef and cook for 2-3 minutes.

9. Ladle the soup into bowls and garnish with cilantro, scallions, chilis and fresh lime. Enjoy!

KETO SOUP RECIPES

CREAMY CAULIFLOWER & HAM SOUP

Servings: 10

Nutritional Facts Per Serving:
Net Carbs: 4.2 g   Protein: 11 g
Fat: 6.2 g   Calories: 123.5 kcal

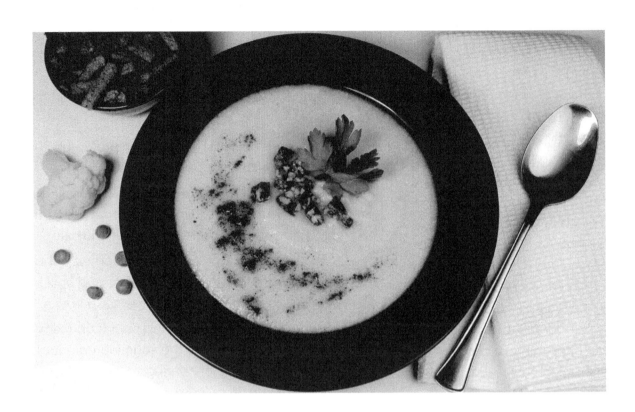

INGREDIENTS

6 cups cauliflower florets
6 cups ham stock or chicken broth
2 cups filtered water
½ tsp garlic powder
½ tsp onion powder
3 cups chopped ham
2 tbsp apple cider vinegar
1 tbsp fresh thyme leaves
2 tbsp butter (or ghee, bacon fat, or coconut oil)
Sea salt and black pepper to taste

This is how you make the recipe

1. Combine the cauliflower, stock, water, garlic powder, and onion powder in a large soup pot.

2. Bring to a boil and simmer for 20-30 minutes, or until the cauliflower is tender.

3. Blend in the pot with an immersion blender (or remove to a large blender and blend in batches then return to the pan) until smooth.

4. Stir in the ham, and thyme leaves and simmer another 10 minutes. Add the butter and apple cider vinegar. Remove from the heat and season with salt and pepper to taste.

5. Serve hot and enjoy!

KETO SOUP RECIPES

CHICKEN FAJITA SOUP

Servings: 8

Nutritional Facts Per Serving:
Net Carbs: 4.2 g Protein: 36.8 g
Fat: 11.6 g Calories: 265.5 kcal

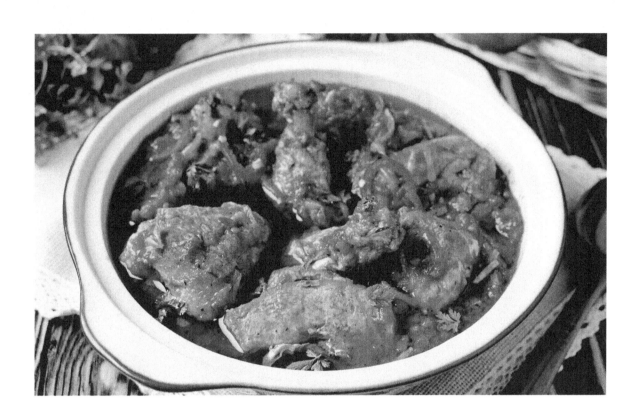

INGREDIENTS

2 ½ lb boneless skinless chicken thighs
8 cups chicken broth
1 can Ro-tel style diced tomatoes and green chilies
1 can diced tomatoes
1 bag frozen small cut seasoning blend vegetables
1 tsp sea salt
1 tsp black pepper
1 tsp garlic powder
1 tsp chili powder
¾ tsp chipotle powder or more chili powder

This is how you make the recipe

1. Pressure Cooker Directions:

2. Place all of the ingredients in a pressure cooker. Seal and cook on high with the vent closed for 25 minutes (I used the soup setting on my Instant pot).

3. Let the pressure naturally release on its own before opening the pressure cooker.

4. Remove the chicken thighs and shred, then return to the pot.

5. Serve with lime wedges, sour cream, shredded cheese, chopped cilantro and avocado, if desired.

6. Slow cooker: Same as above in your slow cooker, but cook on high for 4 to 6 hours.

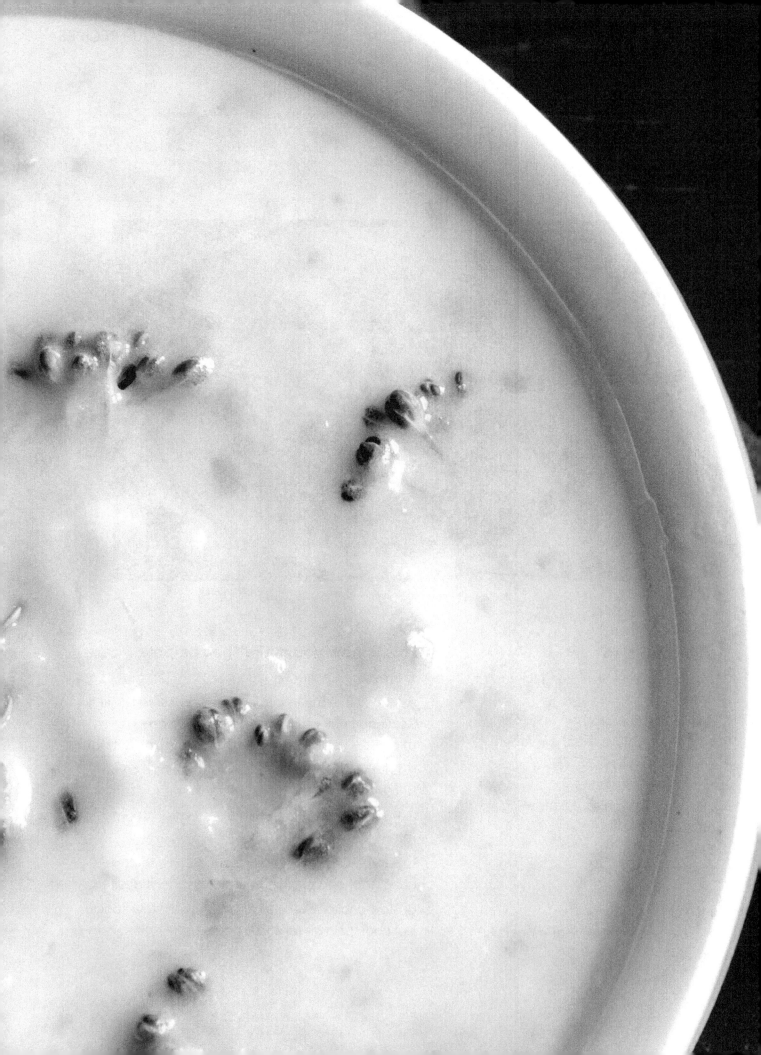

CHEESY CAULIFLOWER & BROCCOLI SOUP

Servings: 16

Nutritional Facts Per Serving:
Net Carbs: 9.5 g   Protein: 21.6 g
Fat: 35.9 g   Calories: 450 kcal

INGREDIENTS

2 tbsp butter
1 medium onion, chopped
5 cloves garlic, minced
Sea salt and black pepper to taste
1 medium head cauliflower, cut into small florets
1 ½ lb broccoli, cut into small florets
1 leek, cleaned and trimmed
4 cups chicken stock
2 cups heavy cream
4 cups sharp cheddar cheese, shredded
2 cups parmesan cheese, grated

This is how you make the recipe

1. Heat a large sauté pan over medium heat. Add the butter, onion, garlic, sea salt and black pepper to the pan. Sauté until the onions are nice and caramelized. About 20 minutes.

2. Heat slow cooker on high setting. Add caramelized onions, cauliflower, broccoli, leek, chicken stock, heavy cream and a little sea salt and black pepper.

3. Mix all ingredients together. Cover and cook on high for 5-6 hours.

4. After 5-6 hours the vegetables will be nice and tender. Using a potato masher, mash up the vegetables. Alternately, you can use an immersion blender for this.

5. Mix in cheddar and parmesan cheeses, more salt and pepper (if desired) and allow to cook 1 additional hour.

6. Serve and enjoy!

KETO SOUP RECIPES

CHILI DOG SOUP

Servings: 6

Nutritional Facts Per Serving:
Net Carbs: 3.5 g   Protein: 3.5 g
Fat: 29.7 g   Calories: 430.8 kcal

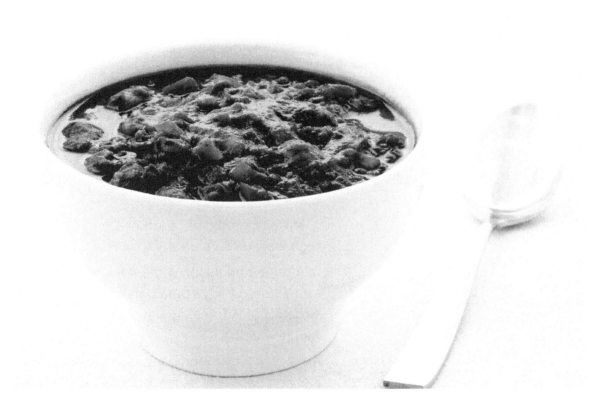

INGREDIENTS

1 ½ lb ground beef
½ cup prepared salsa
3 cups filtered water
1 tsp sea salt
1 tsp chili powder
½ tsp garlic powder
½ tsp onion powder
1 tbsp ground cumin
¼ tsp ground mustard powder
4 good quality hot dogs, sliced
¼ cup low sugar ketchup
2 tbsp Dijon mustard
1 tsp red wine vinegar

This is how you make the recipe

1. Combine the ground beef, salsa, water, salt, chili powder, garlic powder, onion powder, cumin, ground mustard, and sliced hot dogs in a medium sized pot. Bring to a boil and simmer over medium heat for 30 minutes (or 3 hours in a crockpot on low heat).

2. Stir in the ketchup, mustard, and red wine vinegar and cook for another 5 minutes. Serve hot garnished with your favorite chili dog toppings.

3. Chopped onions (raw or cooked), shredded cheese, sauerkraut, cilantro, avocado as suggested optional toppings.

KETO SOUP RECIPES

CRAB SOUP

Servings: 4	
Nutritional Facts Per Serving:	
Net Carbs: 9.6 g	Protein: 28 g
Fat: 63.5 g	Calories: 715.8 kcal

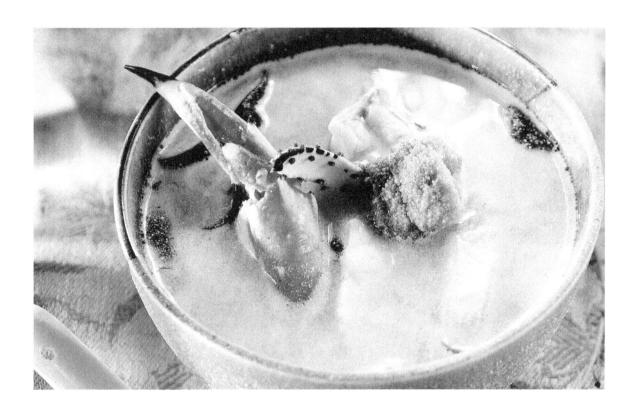

INGREDIENTS

1 lb crab meat
2 cups heavy whipping cream
2 cups milk
6 tbsp butter
1 tbsp cooking sherry
Sea salt and black pepper to taste

This is how you make the recipe

1. Add the crab meat, whipping cream, milk and butter to a Dutch oven or heavy saucepan. Bring to a boil and reduce to low heat. Simmer for 20 minutes.

2. Remove from heat and add sherry, salt and pepper. Serve with lemon wedges and enjoy!

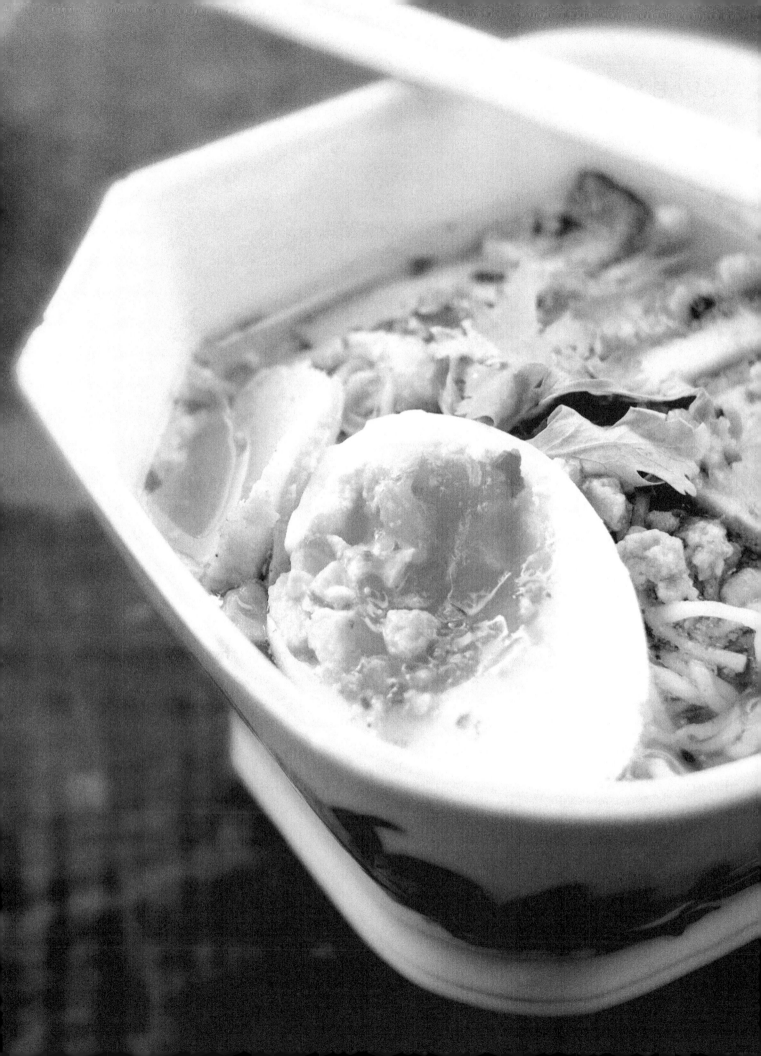

ASIAN MEATBALL NOODLE SOUP

Servings: 6

Nutritional Facts Per Serving:
Net Carbs: 23.8 g   Protein: 27.8 g
Fat: 21.5 g   Calories: 410.8 kcal

INGREDIENTS

For the meatballs:
1 lb ground pork (or turkey)
1 egg
⅓ cup almond flour
1 tsp minced ginger
⅓ cup chopped scallions
1 tbsp gluten-free soy sauce
½ tsp garlic powder
½ tsp sea salt

For the broth:
1 tsp sesame oil
2 tbsp minced ginger
1 tsp minced garlic
4 cups chicken broth
2 cups water
1 tbsp gluten-free soy sauce
1 tbsp fish sauce
½ tsp red pepper flakes
½ tsp sea salt

To assemble the soup:
3 cups shirataki noodles, drained and rinsed see example
2 cups shredded Napa cabbage
¼ cup radish sticks
¼ cup shredded carrot
½ cup chopped scallions
½ cup chopped cilantro
6 lime wedges

This is how you make the recipe

1. For the meatballs: Combine all of the meatball ingredients in a medium bowl and mix thoroughly. Form into 24 bite-sized meatballs and place on a baking sheet. Bake at 375°F for 12 minutes or until cooked through.

2. For the broth: In a medium saucepan heat the sesame oil and add the minced garlic and ginger. Cook for about 1 minute or until fragrant and sizzling. Add the chicken broth, water, soy sauce, fish sauce, red pepper flakes, and salt. Bring to a boil and simmer for at least 10 minutes. Strain the broth to remove the solids and add back to the pan. Taste and adjust seasoning to your preference. Bring to a boil right before serving.

3. To assemble the soup: Place about ½ cup shirataki noodles in a soup bowl. Top with four meatballs, a handful of cabbage, and a pinch of radish, carrot, scallions, and cilantro. Ladle about 1 cup of hot broth into the bowl. Wait about 2 minutes for the ingredients to heat through, squeeze a lime wedge over it and serve.

KETO SOUP RECIPES

BROCCOLI CHEESE SOUP

Servings: 4

Nutritional Facts Per Serving:
Net Carbs: 13.3 g   Protein: 46.8 g
Fat: 74.3 g   Calories: 916.3 kcal

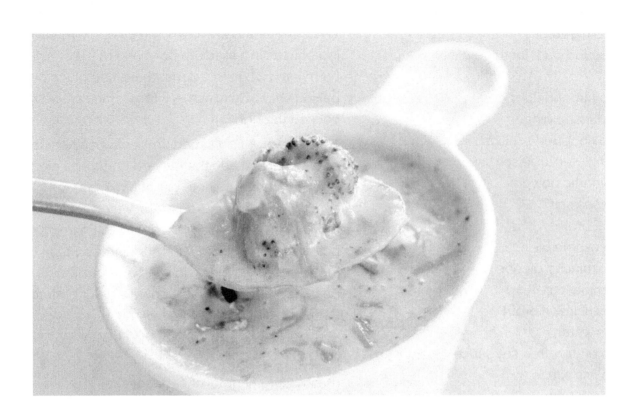

INGREDIENTS

4 cups broccoli, chopped
1 small onion, diced
1 ½ cups vegetable stock
1 tsp garlic, minced
3 cups shredded sharp cheddar cheese
¾ cup heavy cream
Sea salt and black pepper to taste

This is how you make the recipe

1. In a large saucepan over medium heat, stir together stock, onions, broccoli and garlic for about 5 minutes.

2. Once it comes to a low boil, cover and let simmer for 10 minutes.

3. Stir in the heavy cream and continue to cook for 3-5 minutes.

4. Stir in cheeses, until smooth (about 1-2 minutes). Season with salt and pepper, to taste.

5. Serve and enjoy!

KETO SOUP RECIPES

MUSHROOM BUTTER SOUP

Servings: 6

Nutritional Facts Per Serving:
Net Carbs: 4.4 g Protein: 2.7 g
Fat: 19.2 g Calories: 199.5 kcal

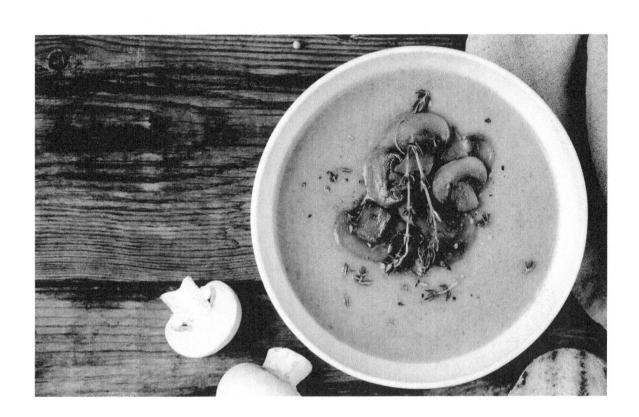

INGREDIENTS

6 tbsp butter
2 tbsp fresh sage, chopped
2 cups mushrooms, sliced
4 cups vegetable or chicken stock
Sea salt and black pepper to taste
½ cup heavy cream

This is how you make the recipe

1. In a large pot, heat butter over medium heat until it begins to brown and turns fragrant, 3 to 4 minutes. Add sage and cook 1 minute more.

2. Add mushrooms and stir to coat, then sauté until mushrooms are tender and lightly browned, 4 to 5 minutes.

3. Stir in stock and bring to a simmer. Cook 4 to 5 minutes more.

4. Transfer to food processor or blender (in batches, if your processor is not large enough). Blend until smooth.

5. Return to pot and stir in cream. Serve immediately and enjoy!

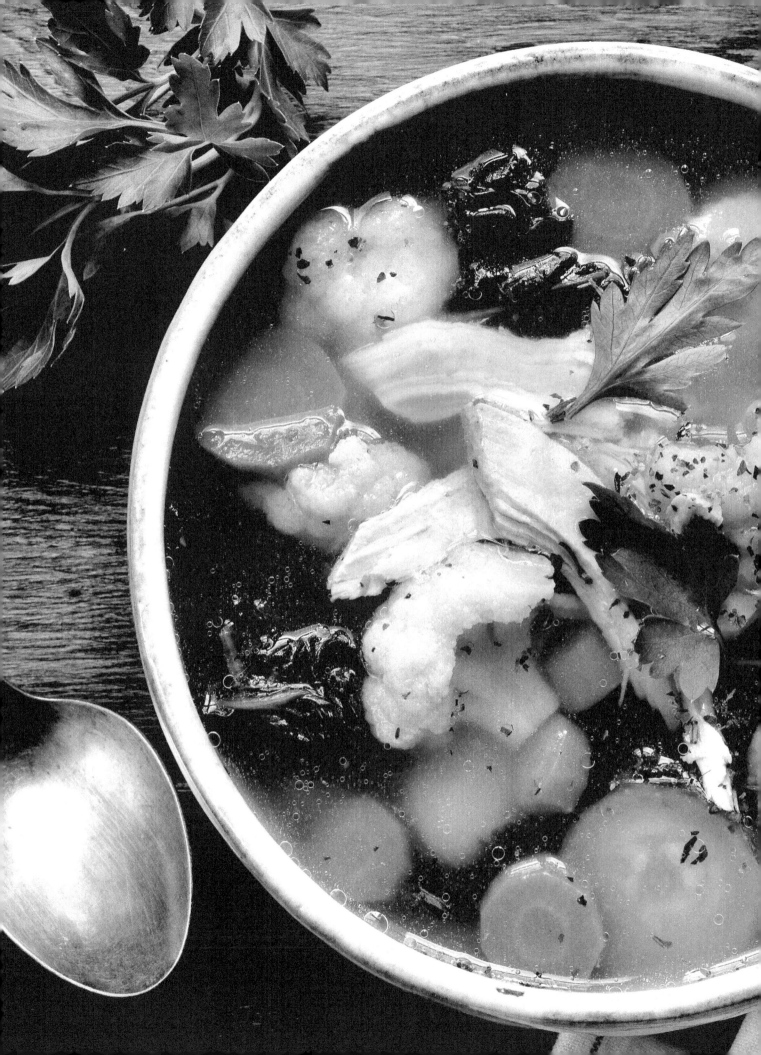

MINESTRONE CHICKEN SOUP

Servings: 6

Nutritional Facts Per Serving:
Net Carbs: 8.5 g   Protein: 30.5 g
Fat: 17.8 g   Calories: 314.3 kcal

INGREDIENTS

¼ cup olive oil, divided
½ cup onions, sliced
1 clove garlic, sliced
¼ cup celery, sliced
¼ carrot, rolled or sliced
1 medium zucchini, diced
¼ cabbage, cut into strips, like coleslaw
4 cups chicken broth
1 can whole tomatoes
1 whole rotisserie chicken meat removed and torn into bite-sized pieces
½ tsp onion powder
½ tsp granulated garlic
pinch of each of the following: dried rosemary, dried thyme, dried marjoram, lemon pepper
Sea salt and black pepper to taste
Pesto, olive oil, parmesan cheese, fresh basil or fresh parsley for garnish (optional)

This is how you make the recipe

1. To assemble the soup, open the can of tomatoes. Chop the vegetables and have them ready to go in the pot group, by group.

2. In a large soup pot, heat two tbsp of oil over medium-high heat. Add the vegetables in this order, stirring them and covering to cook between each addition: Onions, garlic, celery and carrots, cover and cook for 5 minutes, stirring occasionally. Add the zucchini, onion powder, garlic, rosemary, thyme, marjoram, lemon pepper

3. Cover and cook for 1 minute.

4. Add the cabbage, cover, and cook for roughly 2 minutes.

5. Add the tomatoes and their liquid crushing them with your hands, and add the chicken broth and cover, bringing to a fast simmer. Reduce heat and simmer gently, covered, until the vegetables are tender, about 40 minutes.

6. Remove the chicken from the bones of the rotisserie chicken and add to the soup. Stir and warm through. Add the remaining olive oil, adjust seasoning and serve.

KETO SOUP RECIPES

CREAMY CHICKEN BACON CHOWDER

Servings: 4-6

Nutritional Facts Per Serving:
Net Carbs: 8.6 g   Protein: 58.5 g
Fat: 70.7 g   Calories: 903.7 kcal

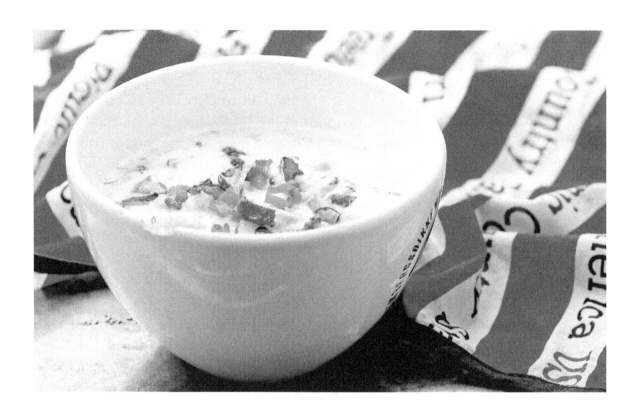

INGREDIENTS

6 boneless chicken thighs
8 oz cream cheese full-fat
4 tsp minced garlic
1 cup chopped onion celery mix
5 cups sliced mushrooms
4 tbsp butter
1 tsp thyme
Sea salt and black pepper to taste
3 cups chicken broth
1 cup heavy cream
1 lb cooked bacon chopped
2 cups fresh spinach

This is how you make the recipe

1. Cube chicken thighs and add to large zipper bag.

2. Add remaining ingredients to chicken in zipper bag. Zip to seal (store in fridge until ready to cook).

3. Pour chicken mixture into Instant pot, add chicken broth and cook for 30 minutes (soup setting).

4. Mix well then add spinach and cream. Cover and let sit for 10 minutes to wilt spinach. Serve and top with chopped bacon.

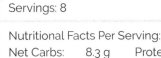

CREAMY MUSHROOM CHICKEN SOUP

Servings: 8

Nutritional Facts Per Serving:
Net Carbs: 8.3 g Protein: 21.9 g
Fat: 13 g Calories: 246 kcal

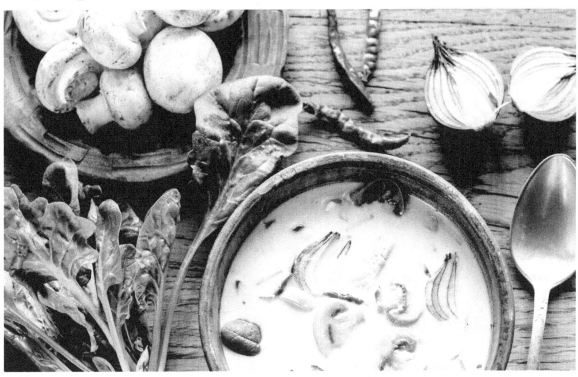

INGREDIENTS

2 tbsp unsalted butter
1 large sweet onion, peeled and chopped
1 cup chopped celery
5-6 garlic cloves, peeled and minced
2 cups sliced mushrooms, mixed varieties
1 tsp fresh chopped rosemary
1 tsp dried thyme
⅓ cup dry sherry
1 lb boneless chicken breast
8 cups chicken broth
⅔ cup heavy cream
¼ cup chopped parsley
Sea salt and black pepper

This is how you make the recipe

1. Add the butter to a large 6-8 quart soup pot and set over medium heat. Once melted add the onions, celery, and garlic.

2. Sauté for 2-3 minutes, then add in the mushrooms, rosemary, and thyme. Sauté until the mushrooms soften and cook down.

3. Deglaze the pot with dry sherry. Then add in the whole chicken breasts, chicken broth, 1 tsp sea salt, and ¼ tsp black pepper. Bring to a boil. Then lower the heat and simmer for 15 minutes, or until the chicken breasts have cooked though.

4. When the chicken is fully cooked, remove the breasts with tongs, and chop into bite-size pieces.

5. Whisk the heavy cream into the soup pot and allow it to simmer and thicken. Stir the chopped chicken back into the soup and add the parsley. Taste, then salt and pepper as needed.

6. Serve and enjoy!

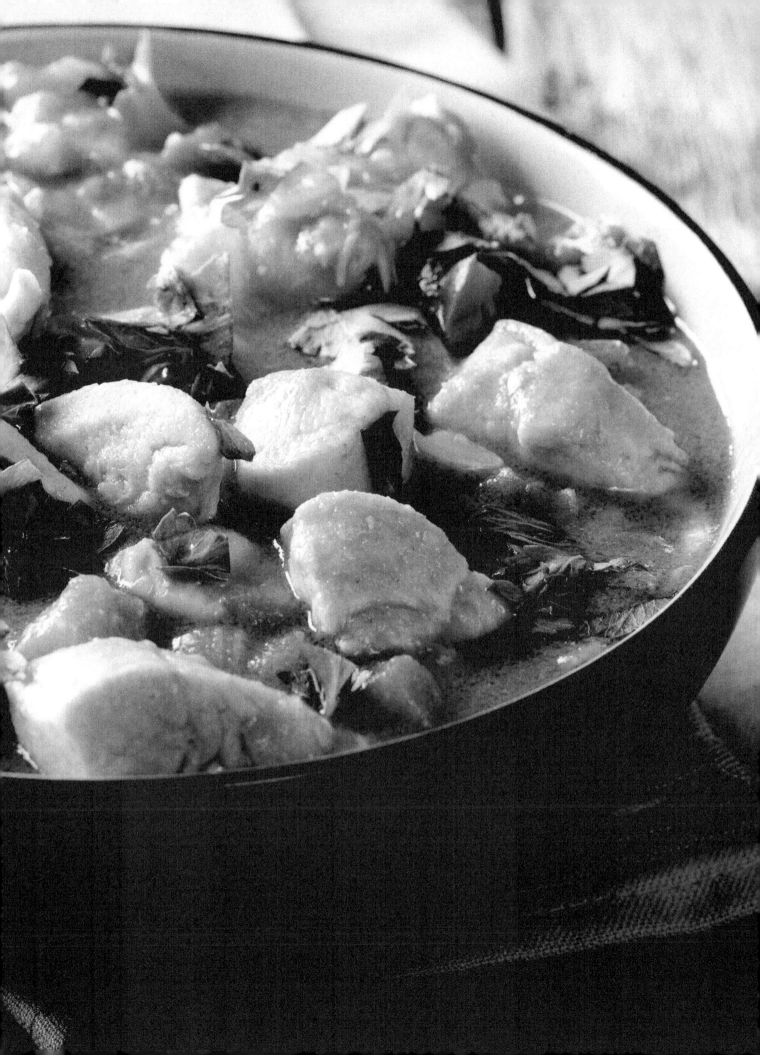

TURMERIC CHICKEN SOUP

Servings: 3-4

Nutritional Facts Per Serving:
Net Carbs: 29.4 g   Protein: 34.3 g
Fat: 22.8 g   Calories: 492.5 kcal

INGREDIENTS

2 ½ tsp turmeric powder
1 ½ tsp cumin powder
⅛ tsp cayenne powder
3 small boneless chicken thighs
2 tbsp coconut oil, ghee, or butter
1 small onion, diced
4 cups of chopped vegetables
4 cups broth
1 cup filtered water
1 bay leaf
1 tsp grated fresh ginger
2 cups chard, de-stemmed and sliced into thin ribbons
½ cup full-fat coconut milk
Fresh cilantro, lemon wedges and red pepper flakes for garnish

This is how you make the recipe

1. Mix turmeric, cumin, and cayenne in a small bowl and set aside.

2. Chop chicken thighs into small bite-size pieces and set aside.

3. Melt 1 tbsp of fat of choice in a medium soup pot. Add onions and cook until translucent, about 3 minutes. Add half of the turmeric spice mixture and the 4 cups of vegetables and cook for another 3-4 minutes.

4. Add broth, water, bay leaf, and ginger to pot and bring to a boil. Lower heat and simmer until vegetables are fork tender, about 8-10 minutes. Turn off heat and stir in coconut milk and greens, allowing the heat to wilt the greens.

5. While vegetables are cooking, heat remaining 1 tbsp of fat in a large skillet. Add chopped chicken pieces and cook until no longer pink on outside, about 5 minutes. Add remaining turmeric spice mix and cook until chicken is thoroughly cooked inside, about another 5 minutes. Discard the bay leaf.

6. Serve into bowls, top with cooked chicken and garnish with fresh cilantro, red pepper flakes, and a squeeze of lemon.

KETO SOUP RECIPES

QUESO CHICKEN SOUP

Servings: 4

Nutritional Facts Per Serving:
Net Carbs: 6.7 g Protein: 33.1 g
Fat: 37.6 g Calories: 491 kcal

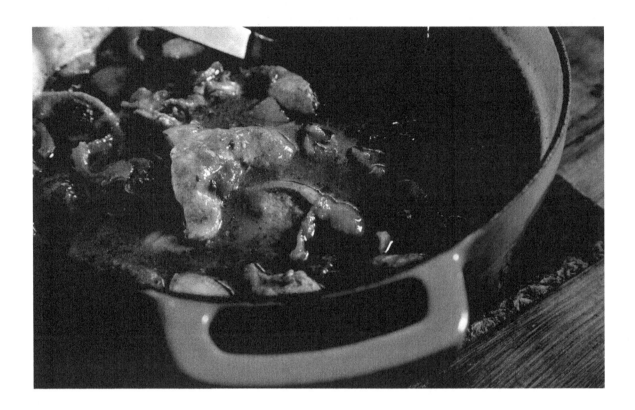

INGREDIENTS

1 lb chicken breast
3 cups chicken broth
1 tbsp avocado oil
2 cans Ro-tel
1 tbsp taco seasoning
8 oz cream cheese
½ cup heavy cream
Sea salt, to taste
Sliced jalapeño, minced cilantro for garnish (optional)

This is how you make the recipe

1. In a pot, heat the oil over medium heat. Stir in the Ro-tel and taco seasoning and cook for 1 minute just to toast the spices.

2. Add in the chicken and broth, cover and simmer for 25 minutes. Remove the chicken and shred, set aside.

3. Stir the cream cheese and heavy cream into the soup. You may want to use an immersion blender to make it creamier than just stirring. Once the cheese has melted add the chicken back into the soup.

4. Season with salt to your taste and serve with desired toppings. Enjoy!

BEANLESS CHILI

Servings: 8

Nutritional Facts Per Serving:
Net Carbs: 10.7 g Protein: 36.9 g
Fat: 16.5 g Calories: 345.8 kcal

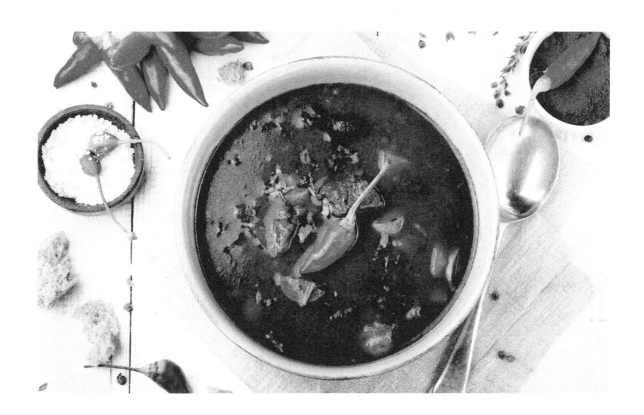

INGREDIENTS

1 tbsp avocado oil
1 lb beef stew meat
1 lb ground beef chuck
1 onion, diced
1 red bell pepper, diced
6 cloves garlic, minced
2 tbsp tomato paste
2 tbsp chili powder
1 tbsp garlic powder
1 tbsp onion powder
1 tbsp cumin
2 tbsp smoked paprika
1 can crushed tomatoes
Sea salt to taste

This is how you make the recipe

1. Heat a heavy pot over medium-high heat. Add the oil and the stew meat. Sauté until browned on all sides. Remove stew meat from pot.

2. Add the onion, red bell pepper, and garlic to the pot. Sauté until translucent.

3. Add the ground beef to the pot and sauté' until cooked through. Add the tomato paste and the spices and stir to combine.

4. Stir in the sautéed stew meat, crushed tomatoes, and salt.

5. Place a lid on top, reduce the heat to low, and let simmer for 2 hours or until the stew meat is tender.

6. Serve the chili with shredded cheese, cilantro, sour cream, and avocado.

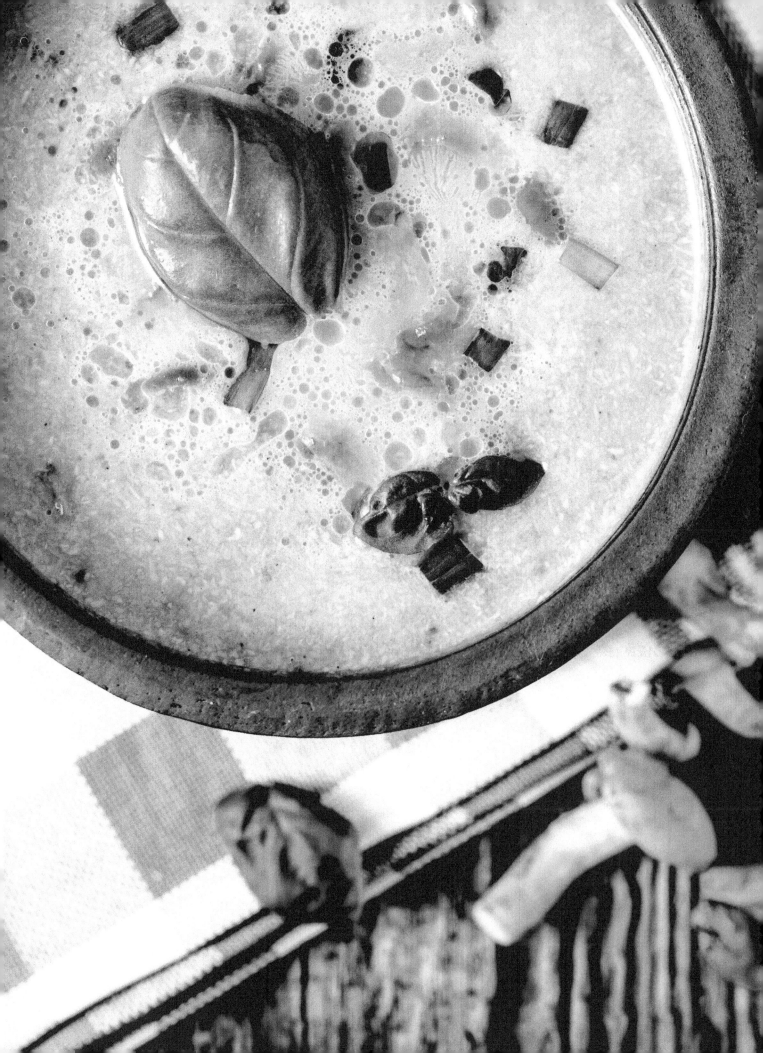

CREAM OF WILD MUSHROOM SOUP

Servings: 6

Nutritional Facts Per Serving:
Net Carbs: 6.5 g   Protein: 4 g
Fat: 30.1 g   Calories: 311 kcal

INGREDIENTS

1 ½ lb of diced mushrooms, combination of white and baby bella
5 oz shiitake mushrooms
¼ ounce dried porcini & wild mushroom mix
1 cup boiling hot water
3 cups chicken stock
1 cup heavy cream
1 tbsp fresh lemon thyme
3 tbsp olive oil
1 shallot, minced
2 tbsp butter
Pinch of black pepper

This is how you make the recipe

1. Add the dried mushroom mix to a bowl and pour the hot water over the top.

2. Add the olive oil and butter to a large pot on medium heat, then add in the other mushrooms and sauté for about 5 minutes. Remove the mushrooms and their juices and transfer to a bowl.

3. Add in the minced shallot into the pot with some olive oil and cook for another 2 minutes.

4. Add in the reconstituted dried mushrooms and the wonderful juices they produced to the pot. Return the sautéed mushrooms back into the pot, along with the most of the lemon thyme.

5. Add in the chicken stock and simmer for 15 minutes.

6. Then add in the heavy cream and cook another 2 minutes.

7. Scoop out a few mushrooms (for garnish) and set aside.

8. Using an immersion blender, purée most of the soup, leaving some chunks of mushrooms.

9. Serve with a few of the mushrooms pieces and a sprinkling of the reserved lemon thyme and enjoy!

SPICY CHILI CON CARNE

Servings: 7

Nutritional Facts Per Serving:
Net Carbs: 11.4 g Protein: 46.7 g
Fat: 38.9 g Calories: 597.3 kcal

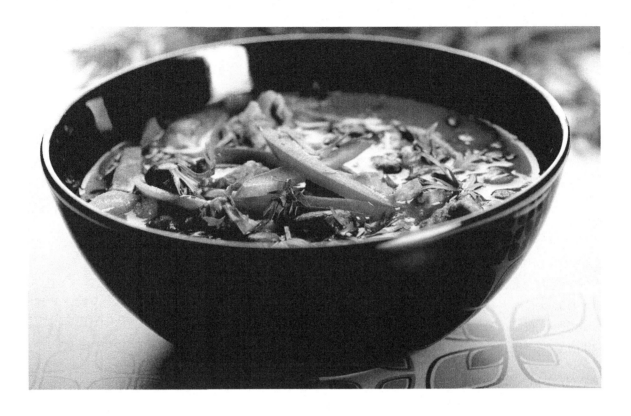

INGREDIENTS

3 tbsp olive oil
1 small onion, diced
3 cloves garlic, crushed
2 small red chili, finely chopped
1 tsp chili powder
1 tsp sea salt
2 lb ground beef
2 tbsp tomato paste
1 tbsp paprika
1 tbsp cumin ground
1 tbsp coriander ground
1 lb canned diced tomatoes
½ tsp black pepper

This is how you make the recipe

1. Place a large saucepan over high heat.

2. Add the oil, onion, garlic and chopped chilies and sauté for 3-5 minutes until the onion is translucent.

3. Add the chili powder and salt and stir well.

4. Add the ground beef. Stir continuously to break apart the meat, sauté for 10 minutes until the beef is well browned.

5. Add the tomato paste, paprika, cumin and coriander and stir well.

6. Cook for 5 minutes before adding the canned diced tomatoes and pepper. Mix well.

7. Reduce the heat to a low simmer and continue to cook, uncovered, for 20-30 minutes.

8. Taste your chili and add additional salt and pepper if desired.

9. Serve immediately and enjoy!

NO-CHOP CHILI

Servings: 4

Nutritional Facts Per Serving:
Net Carbs: 2.1 g Protein: 33 g
Fat: 14 g Calories: 275.5 kcal

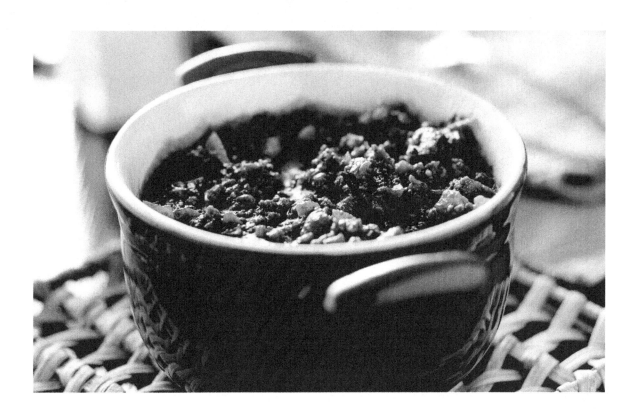

INGREDIENTS

1 lb lean ground beef
1 tsp ground cumin
1 tsp ground coriander
½ tsp ground cayenne
½ tsp garlic powder
½ cup prepared salsa
Sea salt and black pepper to taste

This is how you make the recipe

1. In a medium saucepan, combine the ground beef and all of the spices.

2. Cook over medium heat for about 5 minutes.

3. When the meat is cooked through, add your salsa.

4. Simmer for 5 minutes.

5. Optional garnishes to serve with: red onion, cilantro, avocado, lime, cheese, sour cream, corn, peppers. Enjoy!

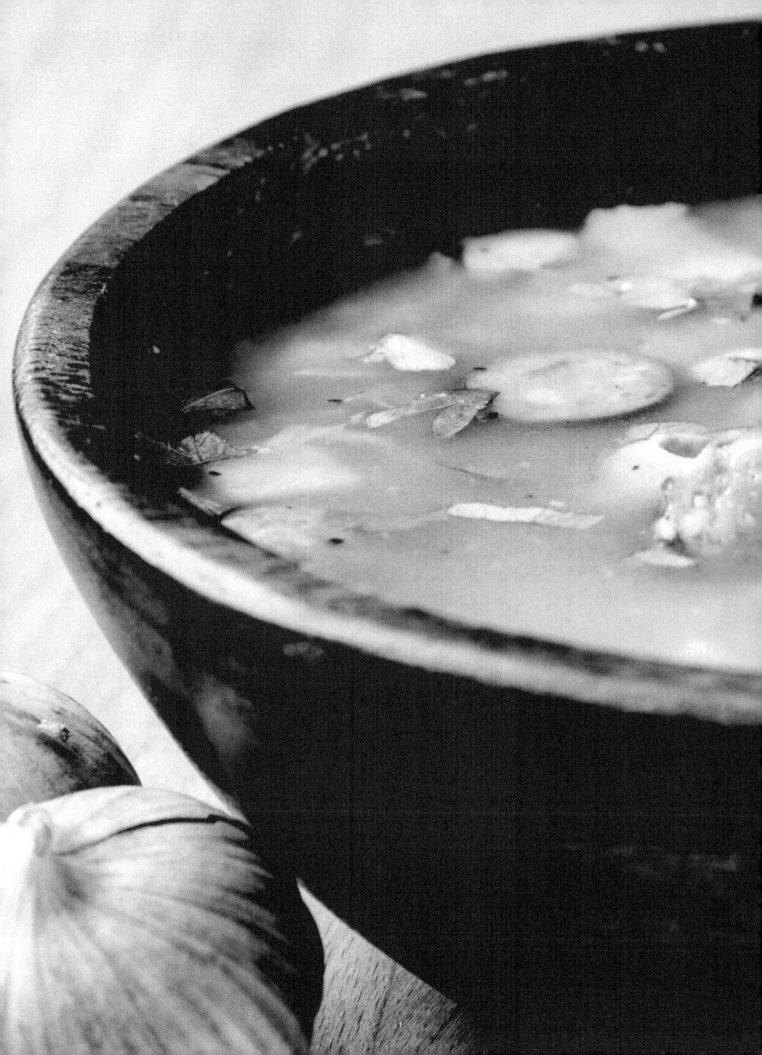

CREAMY SAUSAGE & SPINACH SOUP

Servings: 4

Nutritional Facts Per Serving:
Net Carbs: 5.8 g Protein: 24.2 g
Fat: 25.7 g Calories: 358.8 kcal

INGREDIENTS

2 tbsp organic grass-fed clarified butter (ghee)
1 package organic, fully cooked Italian-style chicken sausage, sliced
1 medium onion, diced
4 cloves garlic, crushed
3½ cups organic chicken bone broth
½ teaspoon red pepper flakes, crushed
6 cups baby spinach
½ cup heavy whipping cream
Sea salt and black pepper, to taste
Fresh lemon wedges, to squeeze on top (optional)

This is how you make the recipe

1. Heat the ghee in a 3-quart saucepan over medium to medium-high heat. Add the sausage and onion. Cook until the sausage is starting to brown and the onion is softened (about 6 to 8 minutes). Then add garlic and cook 1 minute more, stirring constantly.

2. Add the bone broth and crushed red pepper flakes. Bring up to a boil and then cover the saucepan. Turn the heat down to simmer, and cook for another 5 minutes.

3. Stir in the spinach and cook until wilted, stirring constantly, about 1 to 2 minutes. Turn off the heat and stir in the cream.

4. Taste and season with sea salt and black pepper as desired.

5. Serve with fresh lemon wedges to squeeze into the soup if desired.

KETO SOUP RECIPES

BEEF STEW

Servings: 18

Nutritional Facts Per Serving:
Net Carbs: 7 g Protein: 29 g
Fat: 23.9 g Calories: 373.9 kcal

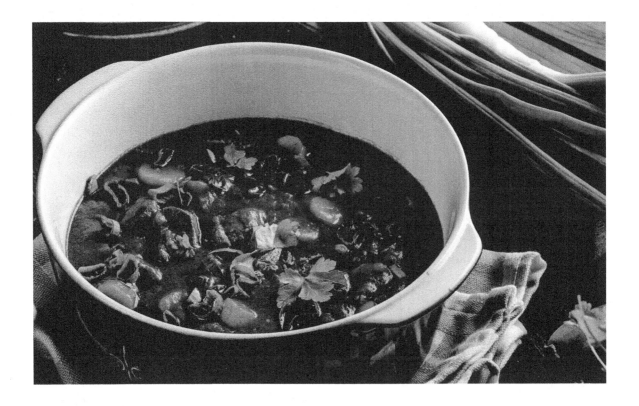

INGREDIENTS

4 lb beef, cubed
5 tbsp olive oil
29 oz beef stock
28 oz diced tomatoes
2 medium bell peppers, chopped
8 oz mushrooms, chopped
6 ribs celery, chopped
4 large carrots, chopped
4 turnips quartered
4 tbsp tomato paste
4 tbsp Worcestershire sauce
1 tbsp sea salt
1 tbsp black pepper
2 tbsp garlic powder
1 tbsp onion powder
1 tbsp dried oregano
2 tbsp xanthan gum

This is how you make the recipe

1. Add oil to a slow cooker and brown beef on all sides.

2. Meanwhile add all ingredients except xanthan gum to the slow cooker. Add beef once it finishes browning. Cover and cook on low for 8 hours.

3. After 8 hours remove two cups of the liquid from the slow cooker and add the xanthan gum to the liquid. Blend really well.

4. Slowly stir it into the beef stew until it's all mixed in.

5. Serve and enjoy!

KETO SOUP RECIPES

MUSSEL CHOWDER

Servings: 4

Nutritional Facts Per Serving:
Net Carbs: 12 g Protein: 19 g
Fat: 65 g Calories: 708 kcal

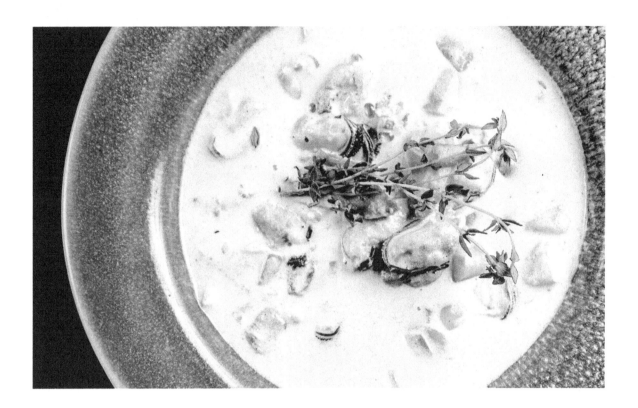

INGREDIENTS

2 tbsp butter
5 ⅓ oz bacon or pancetta
2 garlic cloves, finely chopped
1 yellow onion, finely chopped
8 oz celery root, diced
1 cup filtered water
1 tbsp white wine vinegar
2 cups heavy whipping cream
1 tbsp fresh thyme, finely chopped
1 bay leaf
1 fish bouillon cube
8 oz canned mussels
Sea salt and black pepper
Fresh thyme for garnish (optional)

This is how you make the recipe

1. Peel and finely chop garlic and onion. Peel and dice the celery root.

2. Fry pancetta or bacon in butter until it's really crispy. Remove the bacon from the pan, but leave the fat.

3. Sauté the vegetables in the same pan for a few minutes until golden. Add thyme and bay leaf.

4. Add water, bouillon, heavy cream, vinegar and the mussel juice (optional). Bring to a boil, lower the heat and let simmer for 10 minutes.

5. Pepper and salt to taste. Add the mussels and let simmer for a few minutes. Discard the bay leaf.

6. Serve with finely chopped thyme/parsley and the fried bacon. Enjoy!

BROCCOLI & CHEESE SOUP

Servings: 12

Nutritional Facts Per Serving:
Net Carbs: 5.6 g Protein: 10.2 g
Fat: 24.9 g Calories: 288.4 kcal

INGREDIENTS

2 cups water
2 cups of chicken broth
5 cups fresh broccoli florets
8 oz softened cream cheese
1 cup whipping cream
½ cup parmesan cheese
2 ½ cups shredded cheddar cheese
2 tbsp of softened unsalted butter
Pinch of thyme
Sea salt and black pepper to taste

This is how you make the recipe

1. Cut the broccoli into small florets and set aside.

2. In the crock pot add the butter, softened cream cheese, whipping cream, chicken broth, water and mix well.

3. Once fully combined add the parmesan cheese.

4. Next add the chopped broccoli and thyme.

5. Cover and cook on low for 3 hours or medium-high for 80 minutes.

6. Then simply give the soup a good stir and then add the 2 ½ cups of shredded cheddar cheese.

7. Stir a few times allowing the cheddar cheese to melt completely.

8. At this point you should taste and add the salt and pepper to taste.

Note that this is a thick soup, you can thin it out by adding more water or chicken broth once it is all fully combined.

KETO SOUP RECIPES

GREEN GAZPACHO

Servings: 4

Nutritional Facts Per Serving:
Net Carbs: 6.9 g   Protein: 3.75 g
Fat: 21.75 g   Calories: 234.25 kcal

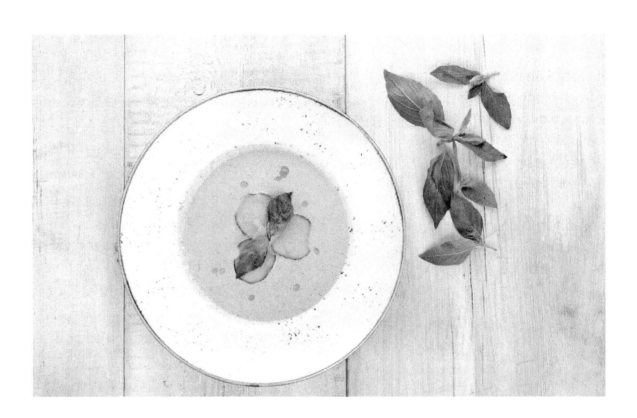

INGREDIENTS

½ cup pre-soaked cashew nuts, drained
½ cup diced celery stalks
½ cup watercress leaves
½ cup sliced cucumber, peeled and seeded
5 oz romaine lettuce (5 large, crisp leaves)
¼ cup olive oil
1 garlic clove
1 tsp sea salt
1 cup chicken or vegetable broth

This is how you make the recipe

1. Combine all of the ingredients in a blender and blend until smooth and creamy. Enjoy right away.

2. Tip! Soaking the cashews in water with a pinch of sea salt for 3 hours minimized the phytic acid in them, making them easier to digest.

3. If you can't eat cashews, use half of a ripe avocado instead.

4. Serve and enjoy!

KETO SOUP RECIPES

SPICY TURKEY SOUP

Servings: 4

Nutritional Facts Per Serving:
Net Carbs: 11 g Protein: 17 g
Fat: 8 g Calories: 186 kcal

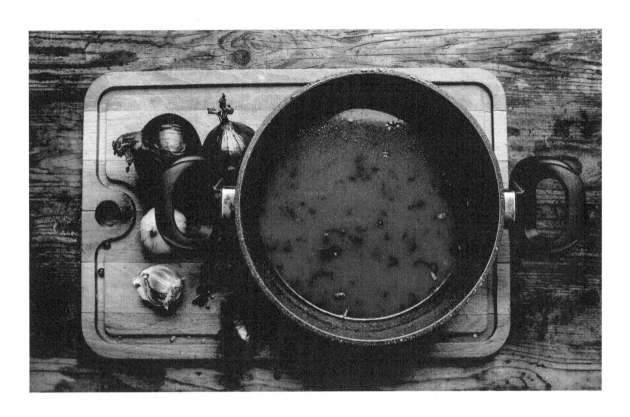

INGREDIENTS

1 tbsp ghee or coconut oil
½ cup red onions, chopped
3 garlic cloves, smashed
1 fresh jalapeño, seeded and diced, plus more for garnish if desired
4 oz canned green chili peppers, chopped
2 tsp ground cumin
1 tsp dried oregano
1 tsp ground cayenne pepper
2 cups tomato sauce
4 cups chicken broth
½ lb leftover chopped turkey or chickens
1 tbsp sour cream, fresh chives, melted ghee for garnish (optional)

This is how you make the recipe

1. Heat the ghee or coconut oil in a large saucepan over medium-low heat.

2. Add the chopped onion. Slowly cook and stir the onion until tender.

3. Mix in the garlic, jalapeño, green chili peppers, cumin, oregano and season with cayenne.

4. Continue to cook and stir the mixture until tender, about 3-5 minutes.

5. Mix in the tomato sauce, chicken broth and add the turkey or chicken leftovers. Simmer for 15 minutes, stirring occasionally.

6. Serve in bowls and feel free for garnish with sour cream, chopped chives and melted ghee.

Tip! Just skip the sour cream and you've got a wonderful dairy-free dish!

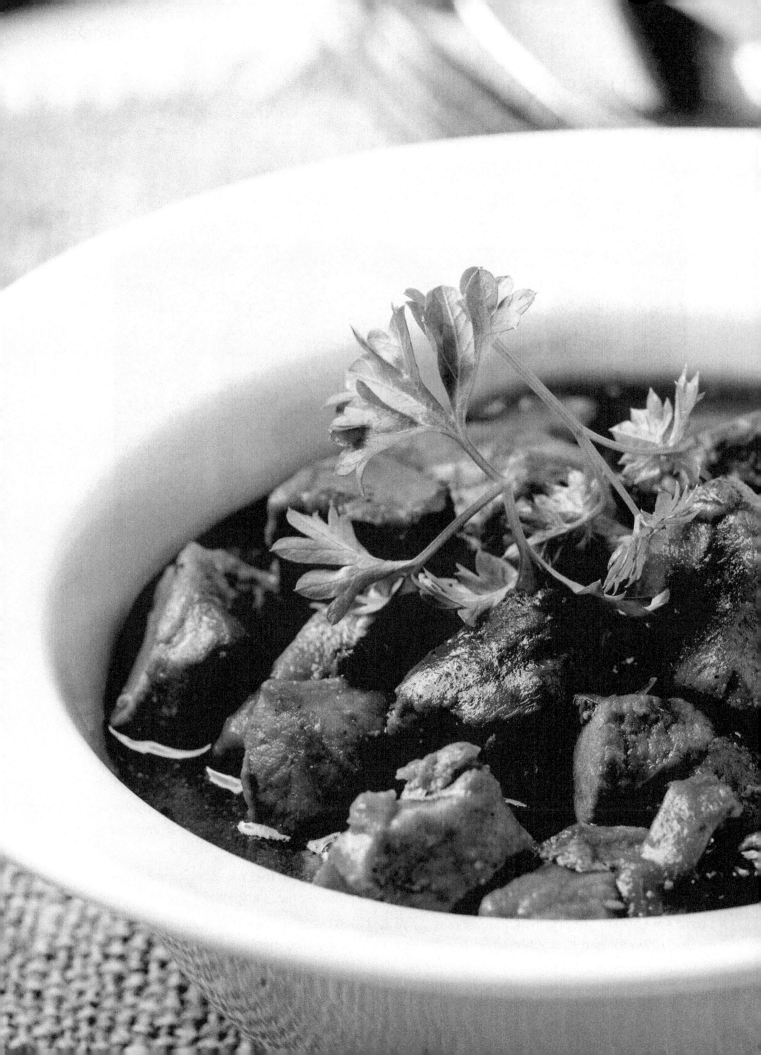

BEEF STROGANOFF SOUP

Servings: 6

Nutritional Facts Per Serving:
Net Carbs: 8.2 g Protein: 47.8 g
Fat: 39.5 g Calories: 588.2 kcal

INGREDIENTS

- 2 large beef rump or sirloin steaks
- 4 cups brown or white mushrooms
- ¼ cup ghee or lard
- 2 cloves garlic, minced
- 1 medium white or brown onion, chopped
- 5 cups bone broth or chicken stock or vegetable stock
- 2 tsp paprika
- 1 tbsp Dijon mustard
- Juice from 1 lemon
- 1 ½ cup sour cream or heavy whipping cream
- ¼ cup freshly chopped parsley
- 1 tsp sea salt
- ¼ tsp black pepper

This is how you make the recipe

1. Place the steaks in the freezer in a single layer for 30-45 minutes. This will make it easy to slice the steaks into thin strips. Meanwhile, clean and slice the mushrooms. When the steaks are ready, use a sharp knife and slice them as thin as you can. Season with some salt and pepper.

2. Grease a large heavy bottom pan with half of the ghee. Once hot, add the beef slices in a single layer - do not overcrowd the pan. Quickly fry over a medium-high heat until browned from all sides. Remove the slices from the pan and place in a bowl. Set aside for later. Repeat for the remaining slices.

3. Grease the pan with the remaining ghee. Place the chopped onion and minced garlic in the pan and cook until lightly browned and fragrant, for about 2-3 minutes. Add the sliced mushrooms and cook for 3-4 more minutes while stirring occasionally.

4. Add Dijon mustard, paprika, and pour in the bone broth. Add lemon juice and bring to a boil. Cook for 2-3 minutes. Add the browned beef slices and sour cream. Take off the heat.

5. If using a thickener, add to the pot and stir well.

6. Serve and enjoy!

KETO SOUP RECIPES

WILD MUSHROOM SOUP

Servings: 6

Nutritional Facts Per Serving:
Net Carbs: 6.5 g   Protein: 4 g
Fat: 30.1 g   Calories: 311 kcal

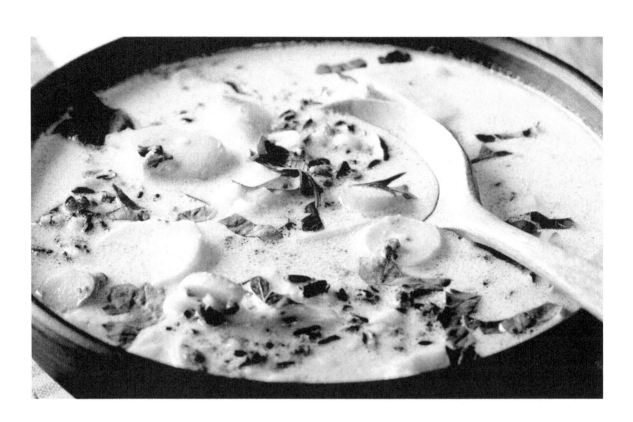

INGREDIENTS

4 oz butter
1 shallot
5 oz portabella mushrooms
5 oz oyster mushrooms
5 oz shiitake mushrooms
1 garlic clove
½ tsp dried thyme
3 cups filtered water
1 chicken bouillon cube or vegetable bouillon cube
1 cup heavy whipping cream
½ lb celery root
1 tbsp white wine vinegar
fresh parsley (optional)

This is how you make the recipe

1. Clean, trim, and chop mushrooms and celery root. Peel and finely chop onion and garlic.

2. Sauté chopped vegetables in butter over medium heat in a heavy-bottomed saucepan until golden brown. Save a couple of tbsp of mushrooms for serving.

3. Add thyme, vinegar, bouillon cube and water and bring to a boil. Lower the heat and let it simmer for 15 minutes or until the celery is soft.

4. Add the cream and purée with an immersion blender until you reach desired consistency. Serve with finely-chopped parsley and a few pieces of sautéed mushroom on top.

KETO SOUP RECIPES

SPICY PORK & KALE SOUP

Servings: 4

Nutritional Facts Per Serving:
Net Carbs: 3 g Protein: 22.25 g
Fat: 39.5 g Calories: 459 kcal

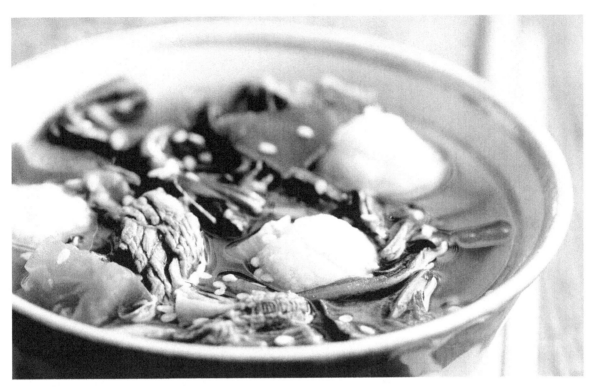

INGREDIENTS

4 oz kale
2 tbsp coconut oil
11 oz ground pork
1 tbsp fresh ginger, chopped
1 tsp garlic powder
1 tsp ground cumin
½ tsp chili flakes
2 chicken bouillon cubes
2 cups water
1 tbsp tamari soy sauce
1 scallion
Savory Asian fat bombs:
2 oz butter
1 tbsp sesame oil
½ tsp sea salt
¼ tsp chili flakes
1 tbsp sesame seeds, roasted

This is how you make the recipe

1. Mix butter, sesame oil, chili flakes and salt in a small bowl. Place in the fridge for at least 15 minutes.

2. When cooled, shape the butter mixture into balls the size of walnuts. Roll them in the sesame seeds and set aside.

3. Heat oil in a large pot or skillet. Add ground pork and fry until golden brown. Add spices and ginger and stir.

4. Rinse and trim the kale. Chop coarsely and add to the pork. Cook for a couple of more minutes.

5. Add water, bouillon cubes, and soy sauce and bring to a boil. Lower the heat and let it simmer for 5-10 minutes. Season with salt and pepper to taste.

6. Serve with finely chopped scallions and drop in a savory Asian fat bomb for flavor.

7. Serve and enjoy!

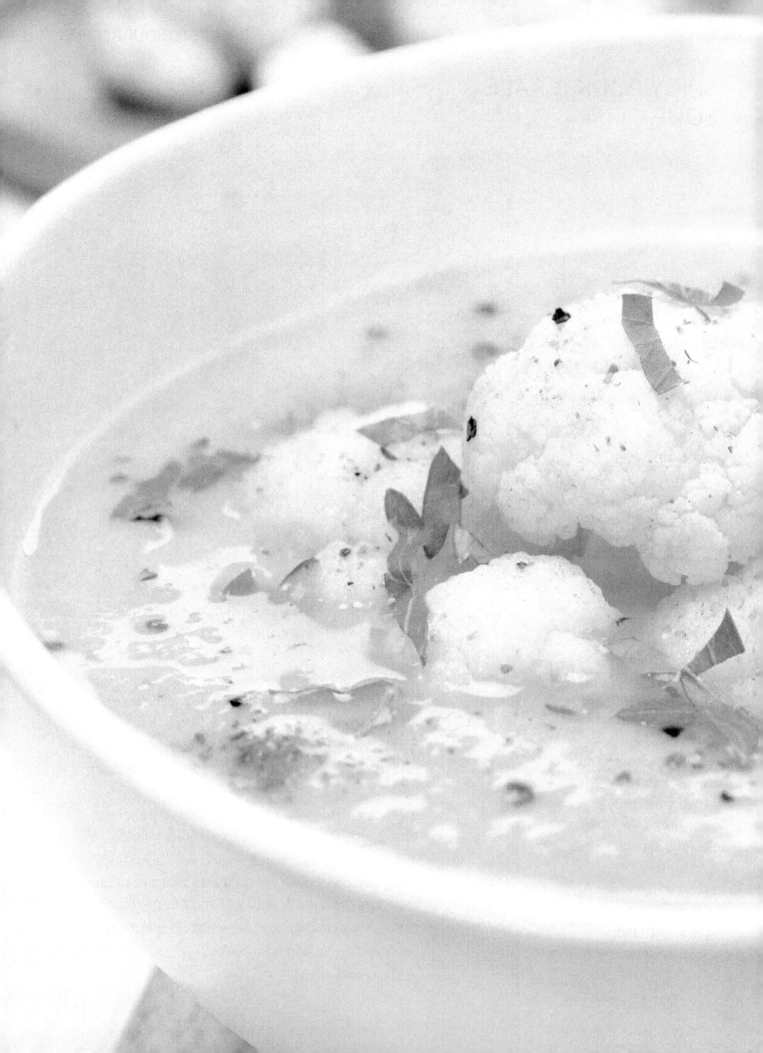

CAULIFLOWER ROASTED RED PEPPER SOUP

Servings: 6-8

Nutritional Facts Per Serving:
Net Carbs: 10.1 g   Protein: 5.1 g
Fat: 5.4 g   Calories: 114 kcal

INGREDIENTS

4 medium red bell peppers
1 head of cauliflower, cut into florets
2 tbsp olive oil
1 medium onion, diced
3 garlic cloves, minced
4 cups chicken stock
1 tsp fresh thyme
1 tsp smoked paprika
Sea salt and black pepper to taste

This is how you make the recipe

1. Cut the red bell peppers in half, scoop out the seeds and lay face-down on a baking sheet lined with parchment paper. Broil in the oven on high until the skin has become black. Remove from the oven and place into a sealed container and allow the peppers to cool down and steam. This step makes it easier to remove the skin from the pepper.

2. Broil the cauliflower florets in the oven on high until they are tender and crisp, making sure to turn them over halfway. Takes about 20-25 minutes.

3. While the cauliflower is roasting, place the oil in a large pot, add in the diced onion and garlic cloves. Sauté over medium-to-low-heat until the onions are tender and caramelized.

4. Add the chicken stock, thyme, and smoked paprika into the pot and mix everything together. Allow the mixture to simmer on medium-heat.

5. Remove the skins from the peppers, dice the peppers and add them into the pot; mix together. Do the same with the cauliflower. Allow the soup to simmer on medium-heat for 20 minutes.

6. Add the soup into a blender 2 cups at a time and blend until the mixture is creamy and puréed. Do the same with the rest of the soup. Add the puréed soup into the same pot, add salt and pepper to taste; allow it to simmer on low-heat until ready to serve.

KETO SOUP RECIPES

CHICKEN SOUP WITH CABBAGE NOODLES

Servings: 8

Nutritional Facts Per Serving:
Net Carbs: 4 g Protein: 33 g
Fat: 40 g Calories: 509 kcal

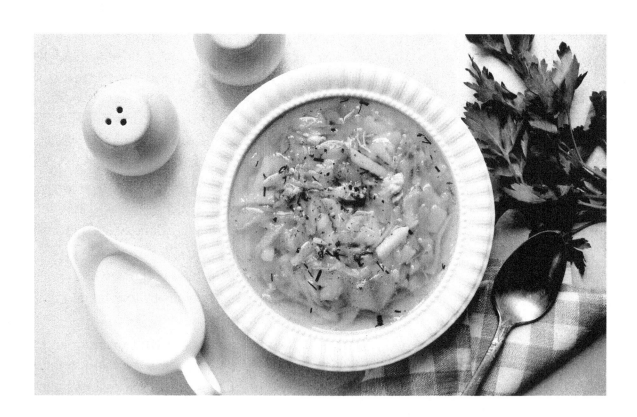

INGREDIENTS

4 oz butter
2 celery stalks
6 oz sliced mushrooms
2 minced garlic cloves
2 tbsp dried minced onion
2 tsp dried parsley
1 tsp sea salt
¼ tsp black pepper
8 cups chicken broth
1 medium sized carrot
1 ½ shredded rotisserie chickens
2 cups green cabbage sliced into strips

This is how you make the recipe

1. Melt the butter in a large pot.

2. Slice the celery stalks and mushrooms into smaller pieces.

3. Add dried onion, celery, mushrooms and garlic into the pot and cook for three to four minutes.

4. Add broth, carrot, parsley, salt, and pepper. Simmer until vegetables are tender.

5. Add cooked chicken and cabbage. Simmer for an additional 8 to 12 minutes until the cabbage noodles are tender.

6. Serve and enjoy!

PUMPKIN & SAUSAGE SOUP

Servings: 4	
Nutritional Facts Per Serving:	
Net Carbs: 6.5 g	Protein: 16 g
Fat: 43.25 g	Calories: 482.7 kcal

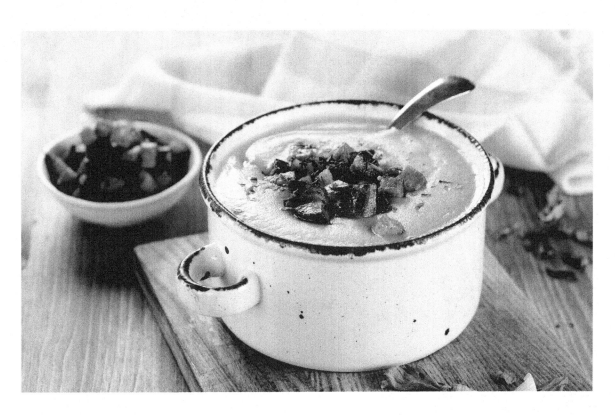

INGREDIENTS

1 lb fresh sausage
⅓ cup minced red onions
⅓ cup diced red bell peppers
1 minced garlic clove
1 pinch salt
½ tsp rubbed dried sage
½ tsp ground dried thyme
½ tsp red chili peppers flakes (optional)
½ cup pumpkin purée
2 cups chicken broth
½ cup heavy whipping cream
2 tbsp salted butter

This is how you make the recipe

1. Use a large skillet to brown the sausage, onion, and pepper on medium-high heat.

2. When pork is thoroughly cooked and the onions and pepper are browned (about 10 to 15 minutes), sprinkle in the seasonings and stir to mix.

3. Stir in the pumpkin, broth, and cream. Simmer uncovered on low heat for 15 to 20 minutes or until the soup has thickened.

4. Add the butter, stir well, and serve warm.

5. Dairy free: If you want to make this soup dairy-free, just use coconut cream instead of the heavy cream and skip the butter. Also if you are avoiding eating pork, you can substitute an equal amount of shredded chicken thighs.

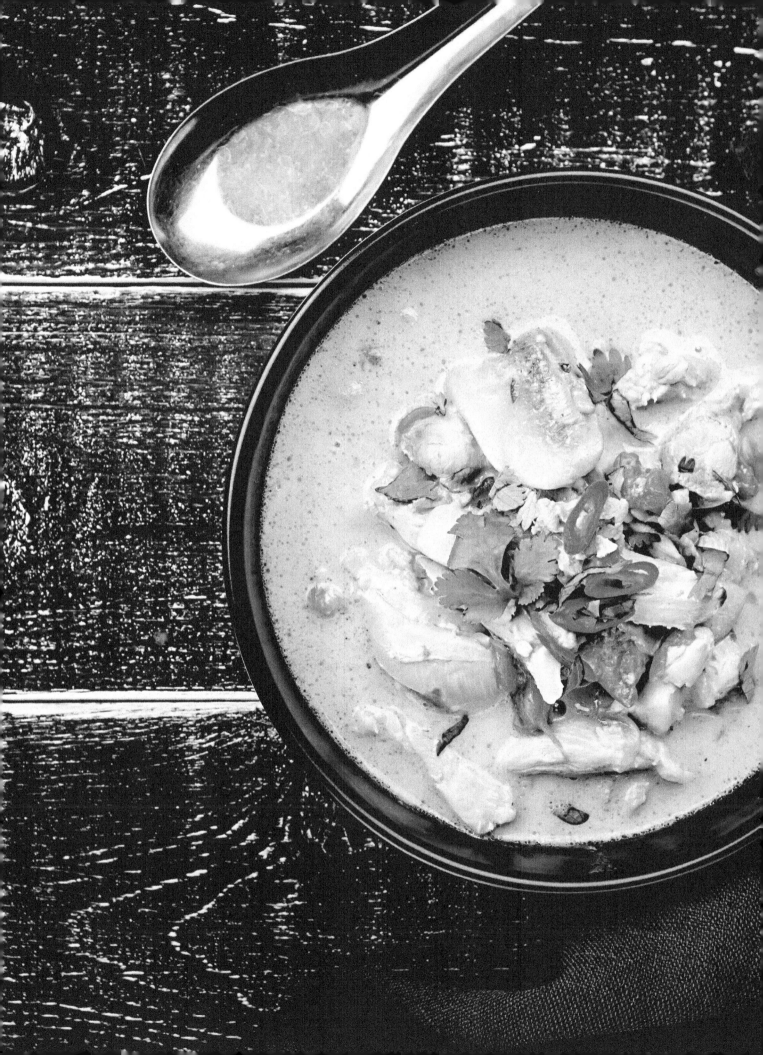

WHITE CHICKEN CHILI

Servings: 4

Nutritional Facts Per Serving:
Net Carbs: 8.8 g Protein: 39.5 g
Fat: 31.3 g Calories: 479.8 kcal

INGREDIENTS

1 lb chicken breast
1 ½ cups chicken broth
2 garlic cloves, finely minced
4 ½ oz can chopped green chilies
1 diced jalapeño
1 diced green pepper
¼ cup diced onion
4 tbsp butter
¼ cup heavy whipping cream
4 oz cream cheese
2 tsp cumin
1 tsp oregano
¼ tsp cayenne (optional)
Sea salt and black pepper to taste

This is how you make the recipe

1. In large pot, season chicken with cumin, oregano, cayenne, salt and pepper
2. Sear both sides over medium heat until golden
3. Add broth to pot, cover and cook chicken for 15-20 minutes or until fully cooked
4. While chicken is cooking, melt butter in medium skillet
5. Add chilies, diced jalapeño, green pepper and onion to skillet and sauté until veggies soften
6. Add minced garlic and sauté additional 30 seconds and turn off heat, set aside
7. Once chicken is fully cooked, shred with fork and add back into broth
8. Add sautéed veggies to pot with chicken and broth and simmer for 10 minutes
9. Mix cream cheese with heavy whipping cream
10. Stirring quickly, add mixture into pot with chicken and veggies
11. Simmer additional 15 minutes
12. Serve with favorite toppings such as: pepper Jack cheese, avocado slices, cilantro, sour cream.

KETO SOUP RECIPES

KALE & SPINACH SOUP

Servings: 4

Nutritional Facts Per Serving:
Net Carbs: 14 g   Protein: 11 g
Fat: 86 g   Calories: 865 kcal

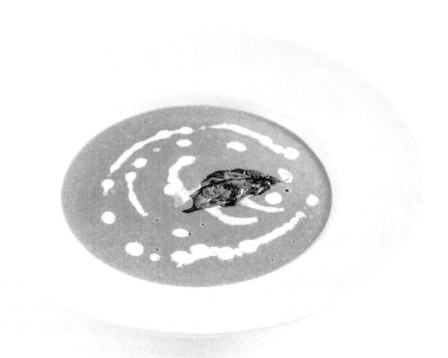

INGREDIENTS

3 oz coconut oil
8 oz kale
8 oz fresh spinach
2 avocados
3 ⅓ cups coconut milk or coconut cream
1 cup filtered water
Fresh mint or dried mint (optional)
1 tsp sea salt
¼ tsp black pepper
1 lime juice
3 oz kale
2 garlic cloves, chopped
1 tsp coconut oil
½ tsp ground cardamom (green)
Sea salt and black pepper

This is how you make the recipe

1. Melt the coconut oil in a hot thick-bottomed pot or pan.

2. Sauté the spinach and kale briefly. The vegetable should just shrink and get a little color, but no more. Remove from the heat.

3. Add water, coconut milk, avocado and spices. Blend with an immersion blender until creamy.

4. Add lime juice. Add more spices if you want.

5. Fry kale and garlic on high heat until the garlic turns golden. Garnish the soup and serve.

PHILLY CHEESESTEAK SOUP

Servings: 6

Nutritional Facts Per Serving:
Net Carbs: 4 g Protein: 29 g
Fat: 24 g Calories: 356 kcal

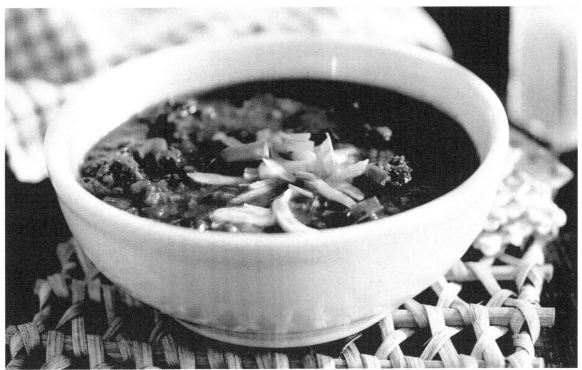

INGREDIENTS

3 tbsp butter
½ red onion, thinly-sliced
1 green bell pepper, thinly-sliced
4 oz mushrooms, thinly-sliced
Sea salt and black pepper
1 lb thinly-sliced deli roast beef, coarsely chopped
4 cups beef broth
4 oz cream cheese, softened
6 oz shredded white cheddar cheese, or other mild cheese
3 oz sliced provolone cheese (optional)

This is how you make the recipe

1. In a large saucepan over medium heat, melt the butter. Once hot, add the onions and sauté until tender but not browned, about 5 minutes. Stir in the peppers and mushrooms and sprinkle with salt and pepper. Cook another 3 to 4 minutes, until tender.

2. Add the roast beef and toss to mix well. Stir in the broth and bring to a simmer. Cook 10 minutes.

3. Place the cream cheese in a blender and add about ¼ of the hot broth from the pan. Blend until smooth and the cream cheese is melted. Pour the mixture back into the pan and stir in the shredded cheese until melted.

4. Preheat the broiler. Ladle the soup into oven safe bowls or ramekins and top with a piece of provolone. Set on a baking sheet and place under the broiler until the cheese is melted and bubbly, 2 to 4 minutes.

5. Serve immediately.

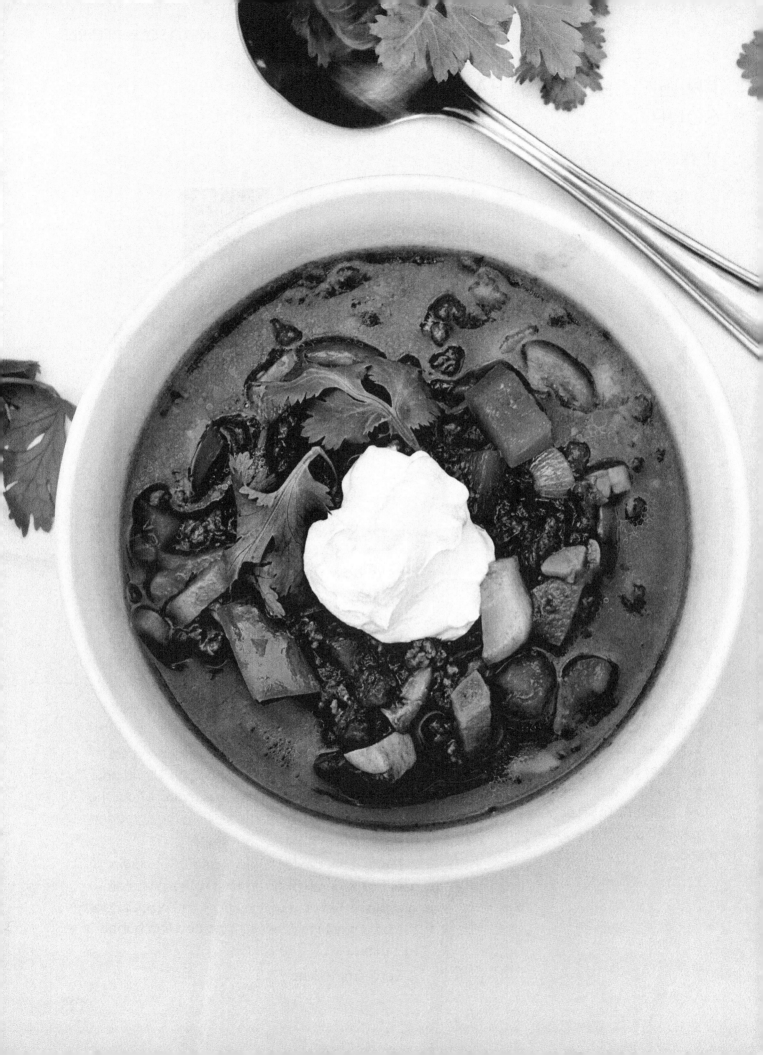

JALAPEÑO CHILI

Servings: 16

Nutritional Facts Per Serving:
Net Carbs: 4.7 g Protein: 16 g
Fat: 5 g Calories: 137 kcal

INGREDIENTS

2 ½ lb ground beef
1 medium red onion, chopped and divided
5 cloves garlic, minced
3 large ribs of celery, diced
¼ cup pickled jalapeño slices
6 oz can tomato paste
14 ½ oz can tomatoes and green chilies
14 ½ oz can stewed tomatoes
2 tbsp Worcestershire sauce or coconut aminos
4 tbsp chili powder
2 tbsp cumin
2 tsp sea salt
1 tsp garlic powder
1 tsp onion powder
1 tsp oregano
1 tsp black pepper
½ tsp cayenne
1 bay leaf

This is how you make the recipe

1. Heat slow cooker on low setting.

2. In a large skillet over medium-high heat, add ground beef, half of the onions, 2 tablespoons minced garlic, and salt and pepper. Once the beef is browned, drain excess grease from pan.

3. Transfer ground beef mixture to slow cooker. Add remaining onions, garlic, celery, jalapeños, tomato paste, tomatoes and chilies (with liquid), stewed tomatoes (with liquid), Worcestershire sauce, chili powder, cumin, salt, cayenne, garlic powder, onion powder, oregano, black pepper, and bay leaf.

4. Stir until all ingredients are well combined. Cook on low 6-8 hours. Discard the bay leaf.

5. Serve and enjoy!

KETO SOUP RECIPES

FENNEL VEGETABLE SOUP WITH CELERY ROOT

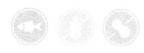

Servings: 4			
Nutritional Facts Per Serving:			
Net Carbs:	9 g	Protein:	2 g
Fat:	36 g	Calories:	371 kcal

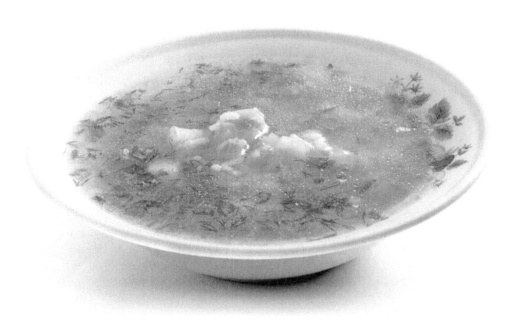

INGREDIENTS

⅔ lb fresh fennel
½ lb celery root
1 garlic clove
2 tbsp olive oil
1 tsp coriander seed
¼ tsp ground nutmeg
3 ½ cups filtered water
1 vegetable bouillon cube
5 oz butter
1 lemon, juice
Sea salt and black pepper
¼ cup fresh dill or fresh cilantro, chopped
10 oz smoked salmon or cooked and peeled shrimp or fried halloumi cheese for garnish (optional)

This is how you make the recipe

1. Rinse and trim all vegetables. Chop finely. The green part of the fennel should be included.

2. Fry all vegetables in oil in a big pot over high heat for a few minutes. Add coriander seeds and nutmeg. Stir and fry for another minute. Add water and bouillon cube.

3. Bring to a boil and lower the heat. Let simmer for about 10 minutes or until everything is soft. Add butter and lemon juice and stir.

4. Remove from the heat and use an immersion blender to mix to desired consistency. Season to taste with more salt and pepper. Garnish with fresh dill.

5. Serve the soup as it is or topped with optional additions like smoked salmon, cooked and peeled shrimp or fried cubes of halloumi cheese.

FISH SOUP WITH AIOLI & SAFFRON

Servings: 4

Nutritional Facts Per Serving:
Net Carbs: 13 g   Protein: 40 g
Fat: 59 g   Calories: 754 kcal

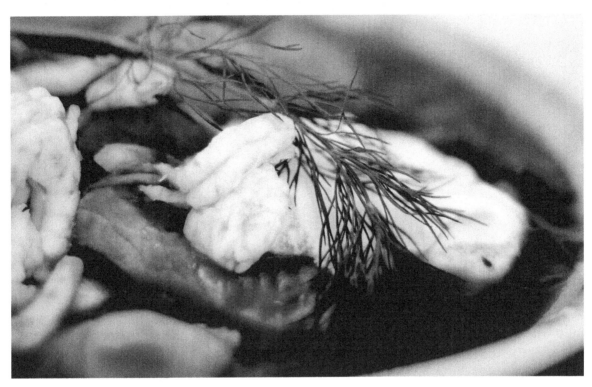

INGREDIENTS

1 yellow onion, finely chopped
2 garlic cloves, finely chopped
1 fresh fennel bulb
½ tbsp tomato paste
1 pinch saffron
2 cups water
2 fish bouillon cubes
1 ¼ cups sour cream
1 lime juice
Sea salt and black pepper
8 cherry tomatoes
25 oz salmon or white fish, cut into 1-inch by 1-inch pieces
Fresh parsley or fresh dill, finely chopped
Aioli:
8 tbsp keto-friendly mayonnaise
2 garlic cloves, minced
1 tbsp fresh parsley, chopped

This is how you make the recipe

1. Fry onion, garlic, fennel and saffron on medium heat until the vegetables have softened a bit. Add the tomato paste.

2. Cut the tomatoes into halves, add to the pot and fry for a few more minutes.

3. Add water and crumbled bouillon cubes. Bring to a boil and let simmer on low heat for 5-10 minutes. Salt and pepper to taste.

4. Add sour cream and lime juice and bring to a boil. When the soup is hot again, carefully add the fish and let simmer on low heat for 5-10 minutes until the fish is cooked.

5. Mix together mayonnaise, garlic and parsley to taste. Serve with the soup.

6. If you don't want to make your own aioli, just use some non-flavored sour cream or herb butter. Sprinkle with extra parsley.

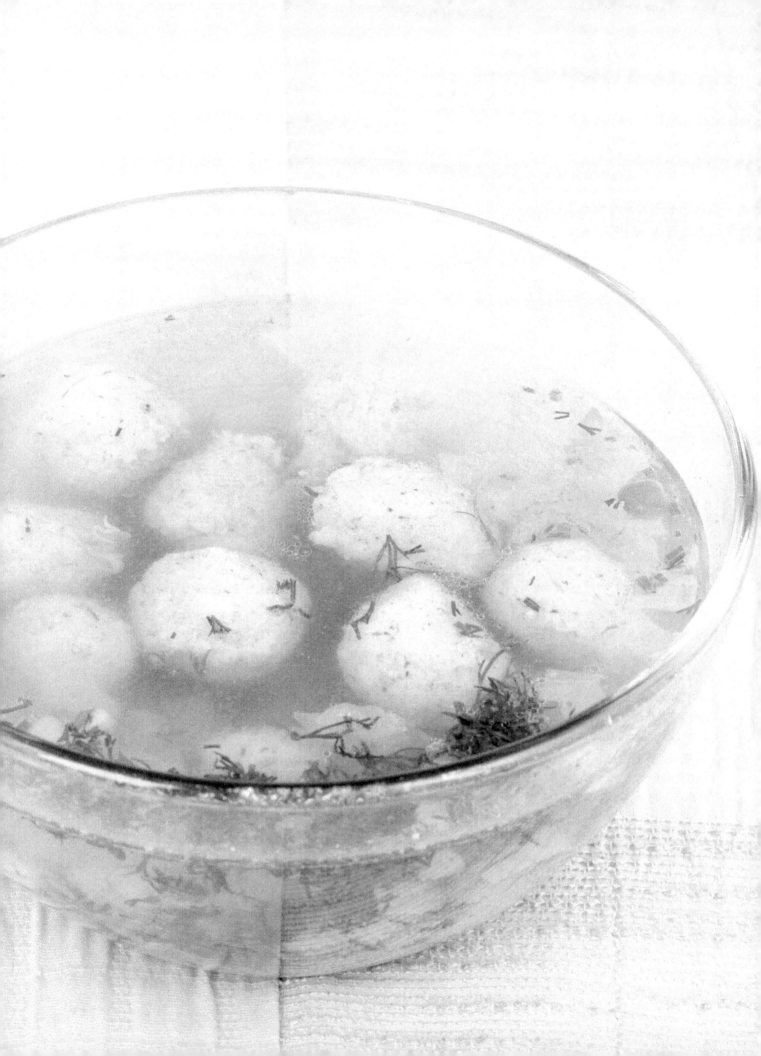

CABBAGE SOUP WITH CHICKEN QUENELLES

Servings: 4

Nutritional Facts Per Serving:
Net Carbs: 4.85 g Protein: 30 g
Fat: 54 g Calories: 619.5 kcal

INGREDIENTS

1 lb ground chicken
1 egg
1 tbsp dried parsley
1 tsp onion powder
½ tsp sea salt
¼ tsp ground nutmeg
1 chicken bouillon cube
4 cups filtered water
1 lb green cabbage or savoy cabbage
2 oz butter
Sea salt and black pepper
Parsley butter
1 tbsp fresh parsley

This is how you make the recipe

1. Chop parsley and gently mix with butter, salt and pepper. Set aside.

2. In a separate bowl, make the quenelles. Add ground chicken, eggs and seasoning and blend until well combined. Place in the fridge to rest for at least 10 minutes.

3. Take the mixture out of the fridge and use clean and wet hands or two spoons to shape quenelles, about an inch in diameter.

4. Shred cabbage coarsely. Add butter to a large pot and fry the cabbage over medium-high heat for a few minutes until it starts to turn golden brown. Add water and bouillon cube and bring to a boil.

5. Lower the heat to medium and add the quenelles, one-by-one. Let simmer for 8-10 minutes or until thoroughly cooked through. Season with salt and pepper to taste.

6. Serve soup with a dollop of parsley butter.

7. You can substitute the parsley with cilantro for more of an Asian take on this dish.

8. Serve and enjoy!

CRISPY PANCETTA CAULIFLOWER SOUP

Servings: 6

Nutritional Facts Per Serving:
- Net Carbs: 6 g
- Protein: 10 g
- Fat: 53 g
- Calories: 534 kcal

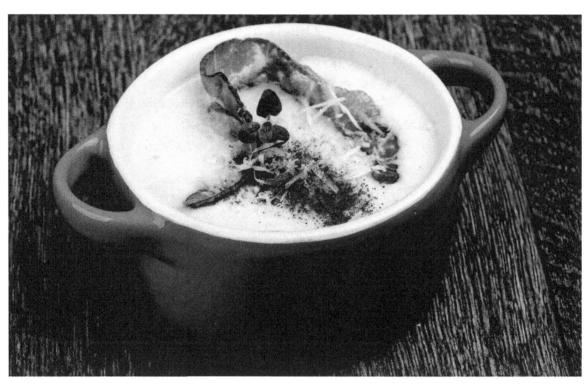

INGREDIENTS

- 4 cups chicken broth or vegetable stock
- 2 cups cauliflower
- 7 oz cream cheese
- 1 tbsp Dijon mustard
- 4 oz butter
- Sea salt and black pepper
- 7 oz pancetta or bacon, diced
- 1 tbsp butter, for frying
- 1 tsp paprika powder or smoked chili powder
- ⅓ cup chopped pecans

This is how you make the recipe

1. Trim the cauliflower and cut into smaller florets. The smaller you cut them, the quicker the soup will be ready.

2. Save a handful of fresh cauliflower and chop into tiny ¼-inch bits.

3. Sauté the finely chopped cauliflower (from step 2) and pancetta or bacon in butter until crispy. Add nuts and paprika powder towards the end. Set aside the mixture for serving.

4. Meanwhile, boil the cauliflower florets in the stock until soft. Add cream cheese, mustard and butter.

5. Mix the soup, using an immersion blender, to desired consistency. The longer you blend, the creamier the soup. Salt and pepper to taste.

6. Serve the soup in bowls, and top with the fried pancetta mixture.

GOULASH SOUP

Servings: 6

Nutritional Facts Per Serving:
Net Carbs: 11 g   Protein: 16 g
Fat: 42 g   Calories: 491 kcal

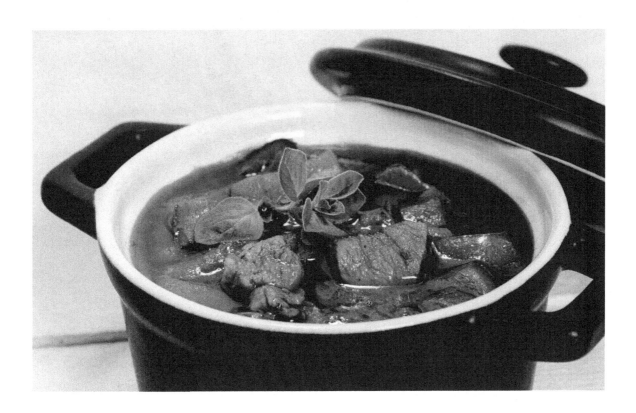

INGREDIENTS

1 yellow onion
2 garlic cloves
1 red bell pepper
15 oz ground lamb or ground beef
½ cup butter or olive oil
1 tbsp paprika powder
¼ tsp cayenne pepper
1 tbsp dried oregano
½ tbsp crushed caraway seeds
1 tsp sea salt
¼ tsp black pepper
15 oz crushed tomatoes
2 ½ - 3 cups filtered water
1 ½ tsp red wine vinegar
1 cup sour cream or mayonnaise
Fresh parsley for garnish

This is how you make the recipe

1. Peel and chop the vegetables finely.

2. Sauté the onion and garlic, with a generous amount of oil or butter, in heavy pan over medium heat until softened.

3. Add the ground meat and sauté, stirring occasionally, until cooked through and browned.

4. Add the bell pepper, celery root, paprika, cayenne, oregano, caraway, salt and pepper. Stir for about 1 minute. Pour in the tomatoes and 2 cups of water.

5. Increase the heat and bring the soup to a light boil. Let simmer for 10 minutes.

6. Add remaining water and vinegar before serving.

7. Serve with finely chopped parsley and dollop of sour cream or mayonnaise.

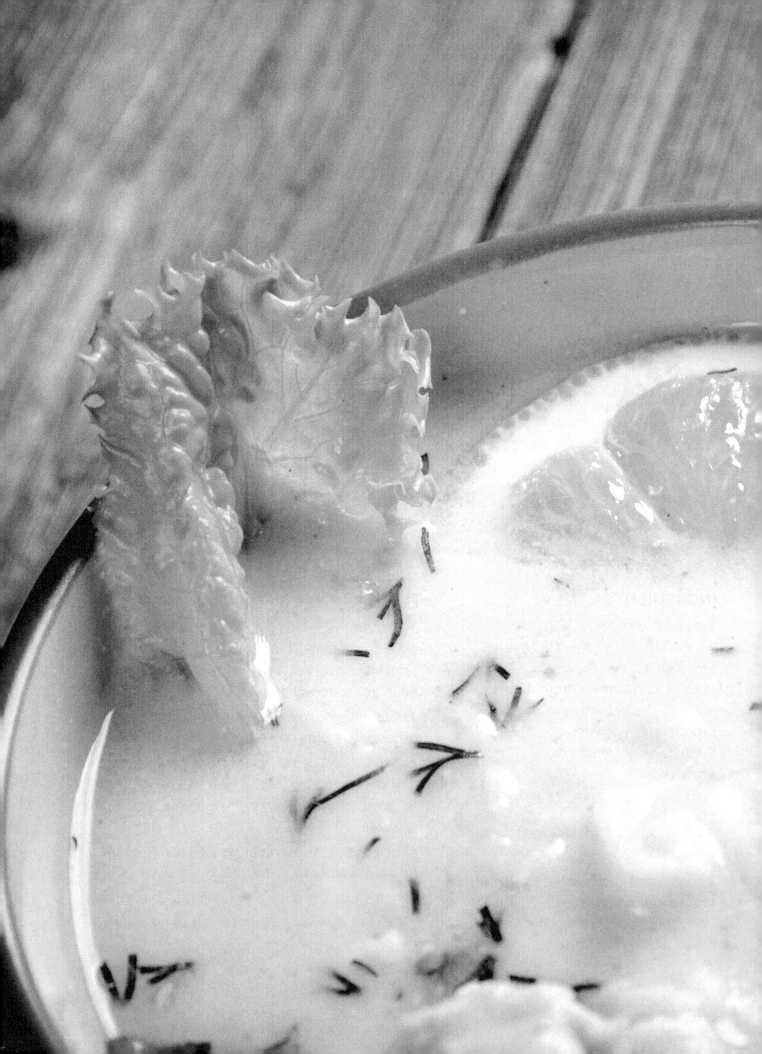

CHICKEN, EGG & LEMON SOUP

Servings: 6

Nutritional Facts Per Serving:
Net Carbs:	2.5 g	Protein:	24 g
Fat:	39.6 g	Calories:	372 kcal

INGREDIENTS

1 lb boneless chicken thighs
4 cups filtered water
2 chicken bouillon cubes
1 bay leaf
¾ lb cauliflower
⅓ lb butter
4 eggs
1 lemon, juice and zest
2 tbsp fresh thyme or fresh parsley
Sea salt and black pepper to taste

This is how you make the recipe

1. Place the thinly-sliced chicken thighs in a saucepan, add cold water and bring to a boil. Add bouillon cubes and bay leaf.

2. Reduce the heat to medium and let simmer for at least 10 minutes or until the chicken is cooked through. Remove the meat and bay leaf. Keep the broth warm.

3. Grate cauliflower roughly (until it resembles rice) and add to the saucepan. Increase heat, add butter and boil for a few minutes.

4. Beat eggs and lemon juice in a bowl. Season with salt and pepper to taste.

5. Reduce the heat and add the eggs, stirring continuously. Let simmer for a few minutes until the soup thickens slightly, but don't boil — it might curdle.

6. Return the chicken to the soup. Serve with lemon zest and finely chopped parsley or thyme.

7. Serve and enjoy!

KETO SOUP RECIPES

ZUPPA TOSCANA

Servings: 10			
Nutritional Facts Per Serving:			
Net Carbs:	7 g	Protein:	14 g
Fat:	19 g	Calories:	246 kcal

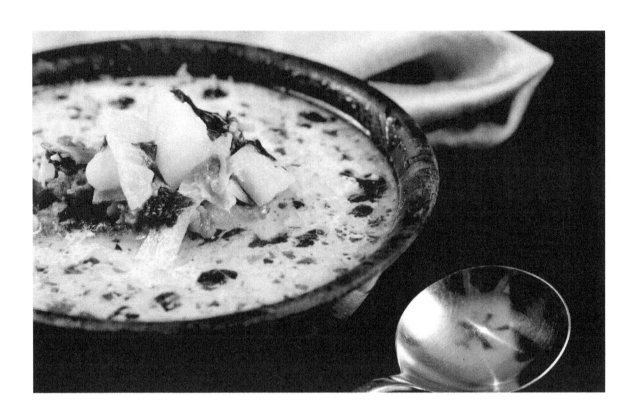

INGREDIENTS

1 lb mild Italian Sausage
4 slices thick-cut bacon
32 oz beef bone broth
1 small onion, diced
3 cloves fresh garlic, minced
1 head fresh cauliflower, diced
½ cup heavy whipping cream
2 cups fresh spinach or kale
Sea salt and black pepper
Crushed red pepper flakes
Shredded parmesan cheese for garnish (optional)

This is how you make the recipe

1. Using a large soup pot or Dutch oven, brown your sausage and bacon together. Cut your bacon into bite-sized pieces to make it easier to cook.

2. Once your meat is cooked, add in beef bone broth, onions, garlic, and cauliflower. Cover and cook on medium heat for about 15 minutes, until the cauliflower is tender.

3. Once the cauliflower is softened, add in heavy cream and spinach (or kale). Cook for about 5 minutes, until spinach (or kale) is soft.

4. Serve with a sprinkle of parmesan cheese and a pinch of sea salt, pepper, and/or crushed red pepper flakes and enjoy!

THAI PORK RIBS SOUP

Servings: 6

Nutritional Facts Per Serving:
Net Carbs: 13.5 g Protein: 13 g
Fat: 18 g Calories: 270 kcal

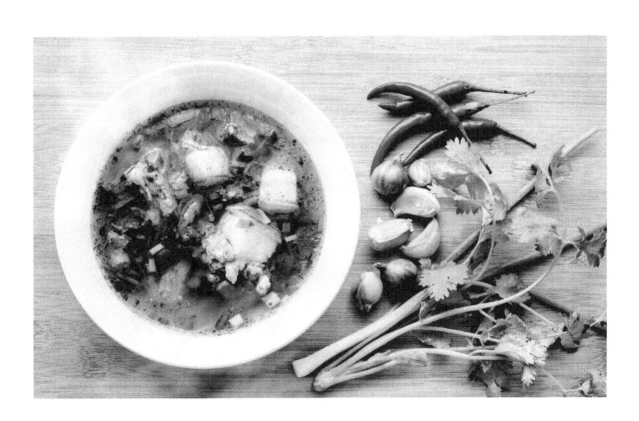

INGREDIENTS

1 lb pork spare ribs (get small ones if possible, cut into 2-inch chunks)
2 small red shallots, chopped into large chunks
3-4 small lemongrass stalks, chopped
10 thick slices ginger
8 cups filtered water
10 kaffir lime leaves or cilantro, tear them up
1 lime juice
2 tbsp fish sauce
Sea salt to taste
Chilies and green onions for garnish (optional)

This is how you make the recipe

1. Place the pork spare ribs into a large pot of water and boil for 10 minutes. Pour out the liquid with the froth.

2. Pour approximately 8 cups of new water into the pot with the ribs. Add the shallots, lemongrass, ginger, and salt to the pot.

3. Simmer on low heat with the lid on for 1 hour.

4. When the ribs are tender, add the kaffir lime leaves, chilies (if you want it spicy), fish sauce, lime juice, and salt to taste.

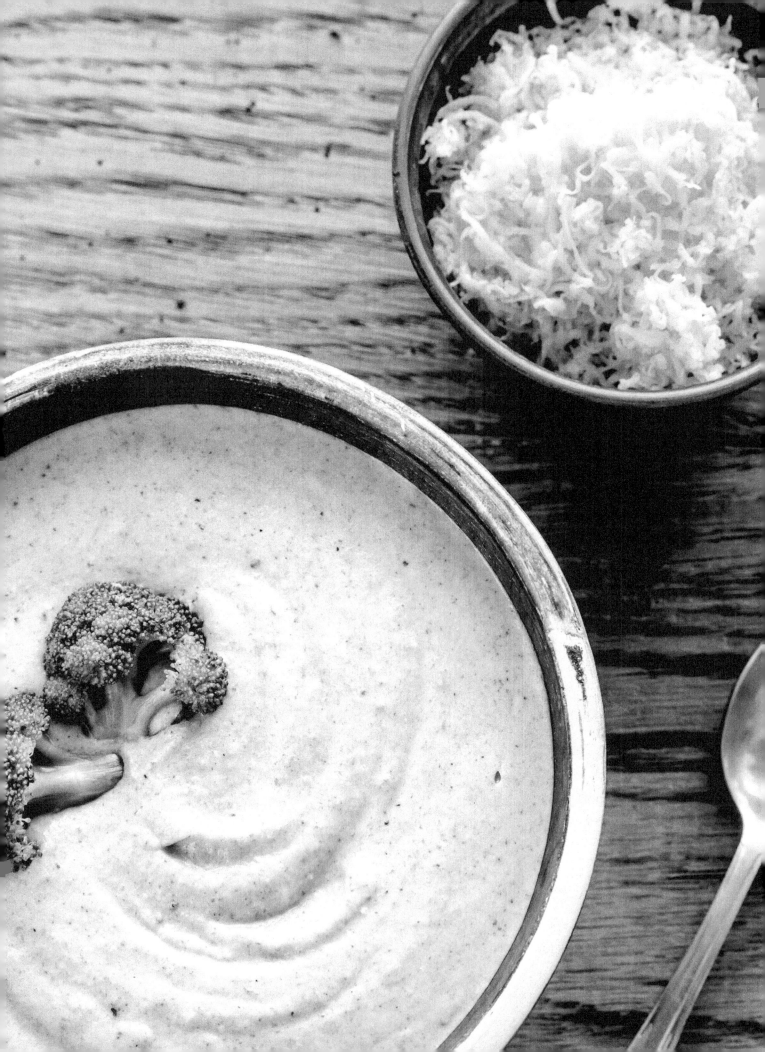

BROCCOLI CHEDDAR CHEESE SOUP

Servings: 14

Nutritional Facts Per Serving:
Net Carbs: 3.1 g Protein: 3.3 g
Fat: 10.1 g Calories: 118.3 kcal

INGREDIENTS

2 ½ cups broccoli
1 tbsp olive oil
3 tbsp butter
1 red onion, roughly chopped
3 garlic cloves, chopped
½ tsp sea salt
¼ tsp black pepper
½ tsp paprika powder
1 pinch cayenne pepper
2 cups chicken broth or filtered water
⅔ cup heavy whipping cream
3 ½ oz cheddar cheese

This is how you make the recipe

1. Clean and cut the broccoli and separate the florets from the stalk. Roughly chop the stalks and cut the florets into small pieces.

2. Heat the olive oil with one-third of the butter in a pot or a saucepan. When melted, add the roughly chopped onion and the broccoli stalks. Fry on medium heat until they start to brown. Add garlic cloves and keep frying until it gets some color.

3. Season with salt, pepper, paprika and cayenne pepper. Combine well and cook for another minute.

4. Add broth and stir well. Cover and cook for 5 minutes.

5. Transfer the cooked vegetables into a food processor and pulse. Slowly add the broth and keep mixing until you get a smooth and creamy soup.

6. In the same pot heat the rest of the butter and fry the broccoli florets. It's best not to move the broccoli around much to get a lovely roasted flavor.

7. Pour the blended soup mixture through a sieve into the pot. For a chunkier soup you can skip the sieve. Combine well and add more salt and pepper if needed. If the soup seems to be too thick, you can add some water.

8. Allow the mixture to come to a boil and then simmer for a few minutes.

9. Add cream and cheese and mix well. Cook until the cheese has melted.

10. Serve hot and garnish with some shredded cheddar cheese.

KETO SOUP RECIPES

BACON CABBAGE CHUCK ROAST STEW

Servings: 6

Nutritional Facts Per Serving:
Net Carbs: 5.1 g Protein: 71 g
Fat: 48 g Calories: 744 kcal

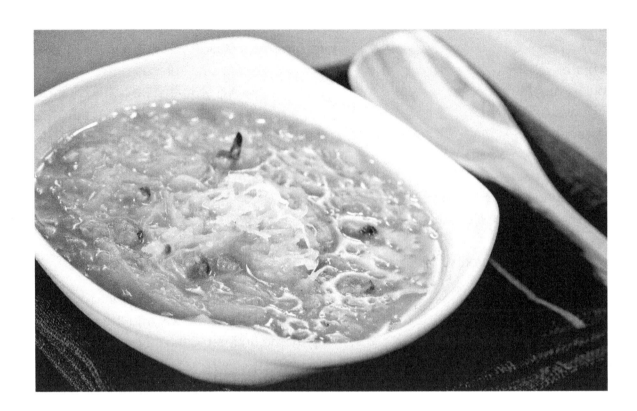

INGREDIENTS

½ lb of uncured bacon, in strips
2-3 lb grass-fed and finished chuck roast, cut in 2-inch pieces
2 large red onions, peeled and sliced
1 clove garlic, peeled and smashed
1 small green or savoy cabbage
Sea salt and black pepper to taste
1 sprig fresh thyme
1 cup beef bone broth

This is how you make the recipe

1. Line the bottom of a slow cooker with bacon slices.

2. Add onion slices, garlic, chuck roast, cabbage slices, thyme, broth, few pinches of sea salt and a liberal amount of freshly-ground black pepper.

3. Cook on low for 7 hours.

4. Serve and enjoy!

SOUTHERN POTLIKKER SOUP

Servings: 6

Nutritional Facts Per Serving:
Net Carbs: 11.4 g
Fat: 12 g
Protein: 23.8 g
Calories: 273 kcal

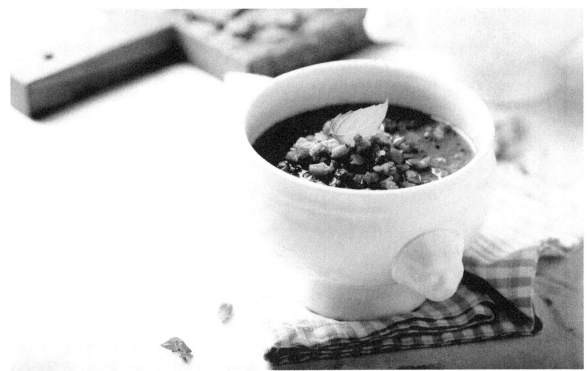

INGREDIENTS

3 tbsp ghee or butter
1 large onion, diced
1 lb uncured, fully-cooked ham steak, cubed
2-3 garlic cloves, minced
2 celery stalks, chopped
2 carrots, peeled and chopped
6 cups chicken or veggie broth
4 cups chopped kale (well-rinsed and middle vein and stems discarded)
6 cups chopped collards (well-rinsed and middle vein and stems discarded)
1 tbsp apple cider vinegar
1 tbsp Sriracha (or preferred hot sauce)
Sea salt and black pepper to taste

This is how you make the recipe

1. In a Dutch oven or heavy-bottomed pot, heat butter, onion, ham, garlic, celery, and carrots. Cook over medium heat and stir until onions are translucent.

2. Add broth, scraping any bits off the bottom of the pot. Add greens, apple cider vinegar, Sriracha, salt and pepper.

3. Bring to a boil. Reduce heat and cover. Simmer for 1 ½ hours.

4. Serve and enjoy!

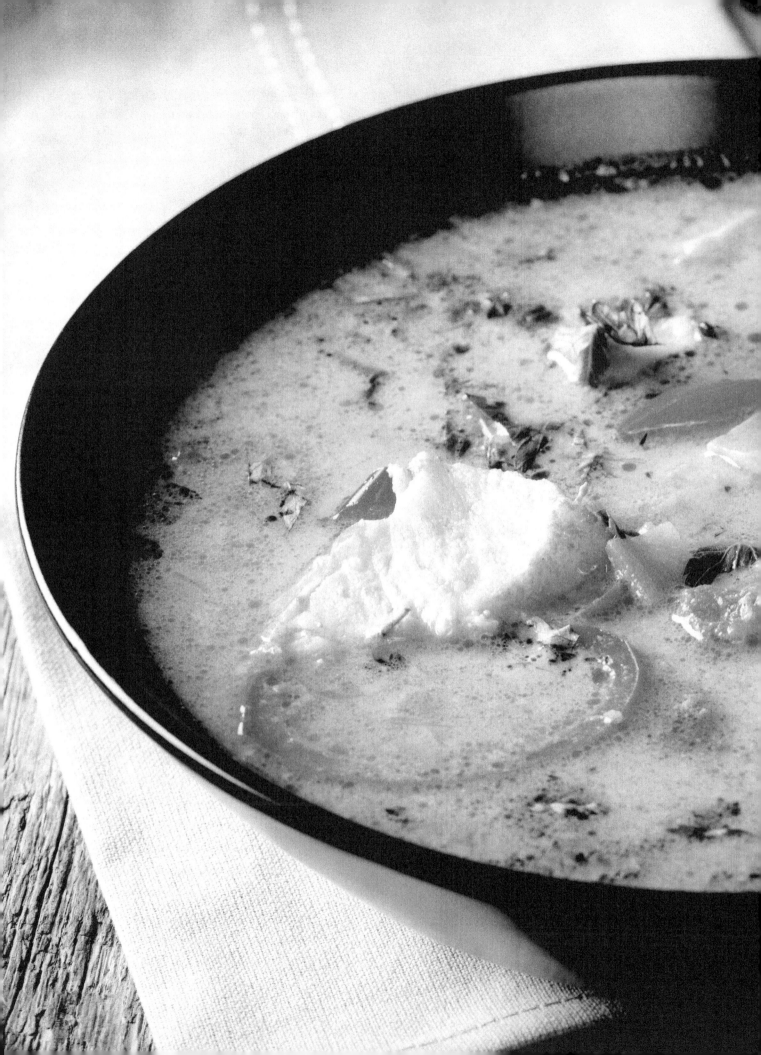

TURKEY SOUP WITH CILANTRO BUTTER

Servings: 4

Nutritional Facts Per Serving:
Net Carbs: 12.5 g Protein: 34 g
Fat: 100.5 g Calories: 1061 kcal

INGREDIENTS

3 tbsp coconut oil
1 yellow onion
1 oz grated fresh ginger
1 lb ground turkey or ground chicken
1 tbsp green curry paste
1 green bell pepper or yellow bell pepper
27 oz coconut milk
2 cups filtered water
2 tsp sea salt
½ tsp back pepper
Cilantro butter:
2 tbsp olive oil
⅓ cup chopped fresh cilantro
4 oz butter
1 tsp sea salt
½ tsp crushed coriander seed
1 pinch pepper
1 tbsp lime juice

This is how you make the recipe

1. Finely chop onion and ginger. Sauté in oil in a large skillet or sauce pan, until the onions are translucent.

2. Add ground poultry and stir until fully cooked. Add curry paste and bell peppers, and stir until incorporated.

3. Add the remaining soup ingredients, except for the beans, and bring to a boil. Lower the heat and let simmer for about 20 minutes.

4. Serve the soup in bowls and top off with cilantro butter.

5. Mix oil and cilantro using an immersion blender.

6. Add butter and other remaining ingredients and whip with an immersion mixer until fluffy. Serve with the soup and enjoy!

ASIAN MEATBALL CHICKEN SOUP

Servings: 2

Nutritional Facts Per Serving:
Net Carbs: 3.4 g   Protein: 34.5 g
Fat: 29.5 g   Calories: 412 kcal

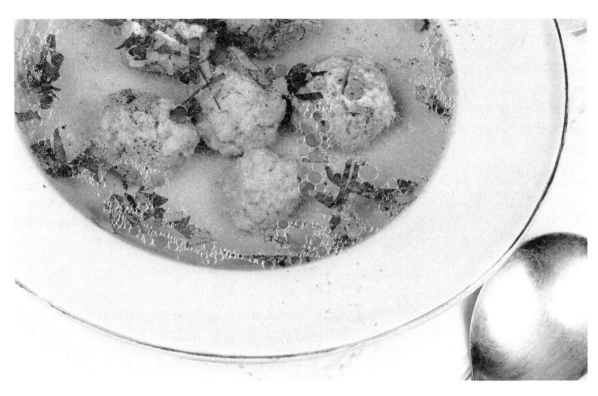

INGREDIENTS

10 oz of ground chicken
1 tbsp of chives, finely chopped
1 tbsp of fresh ginger, finely minced
Sea salt and black pepper to taste
2 tbsp of avocado oil
2 ½ cups of chicken broth
2 star anise
1 tsp of fish sauce
2 green onions, sliced
5 slices of fresh ginger

This is how you make the recipe

1. Combine the ground chicken with the chives and ginger and season the mixture with salt and pepper. Form into golfball-sized pieces and place in the fridge while you make the fragrant broth.

2. Pour the chicken broth into a pan and add the star anise, fish sauce, and ginger slices.

3. Bring to a boil, then reduce to a simmer for 10-15 minutes.

4. Heat the avocado oil in a pan and cook the chicken meatballs until browned on the outside and sufficiently cooked on the inside.

5. Taste the broth for flavor and adjust accordingly with additional simmering (to concentrate flavor) or by the addition of more fish sauce. Strain and divide between two bowls. Add the cooked meatballs into the bowls of broth and scatter over the green onions and enjoy!

HAMBURGER SOUP

Servings: 4

Nutritional Facts Per Serving:
Net Carbs: 5.6 g   Protein: 39.3 g
Fat: 27.3 g   Calories: 434.3 kcal

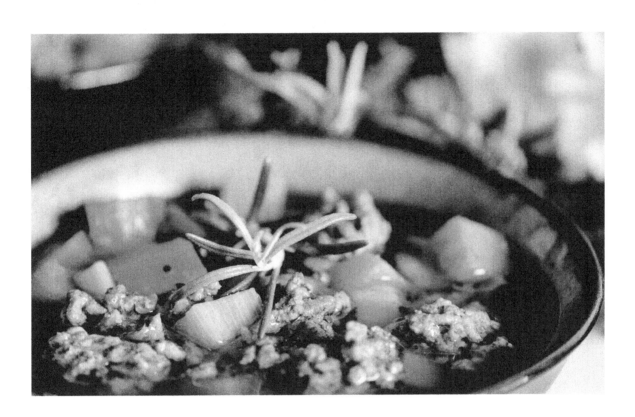

INGREDIENTS

1 lb ground beef
2 tbsp avocado oil
1 carrot, diced
4 stalks of celery, diced
1 zucchini, diced
½ onion, diced
3 cups bone broth
2 tomatoes, diced
2 bay leaves
10 basil leaves, chopped

This is how you make the recipe

1. Add avocado oil into a large pot.

2. Sauté the ground beef until completely browned.

3. Add in the carrot, celery, zucchini and onion. Brown them all slightly.

4. Pour in the 3 cups of bone broth and add in the tomatoes, bay leaves.

5. Bring to a boil, and then turn down the heat and let simmer with the lid on for 1 ½ hours, stirring occasionally.

6. Remove the bay leaves, season with salt and pepper to taste and add in the chopped basil leaves. Then serve and enjoy!

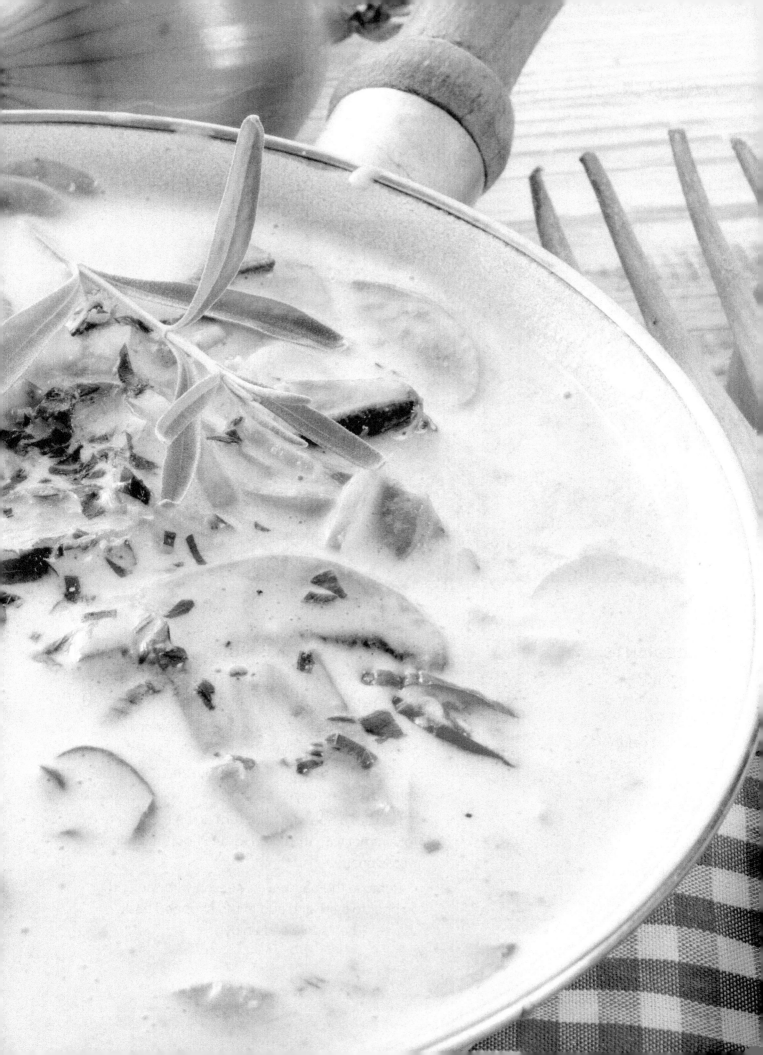

MUSHROOM SOUP

Servings: 4

Nutritional Facts Per Serving:
Net Carbs: 5 g Protein: 15 g
Fat: 95 g Calories: 960 kcal

INGREDIENTS

3 oz prosciutto ham
1 yellow onion
1 lb mushrooms
4 oz butter
1 tsp dried thyme
1 tsp sea salt
¼ tsp black pepper
⅓ cup dry white wine
7 oz cream cheese
2 cups filtered water
4 egg yolks
1 cup heavy whipping cream
Parsley oil:
½ cup olive oil
1 oz fresh parsley
Sea salt and black pepper

This is how you make the recipe

1. Preheat the oven to 300°F, preferably using the oven's convection setting.

2. Put thin slices of prosciutto ham on a baking sheet lined with parchment paper and bake on upper rack in the oven. Check on them every 5 minutes and flip them a few times while drying. It will take about 30 minutes for the ham to crisp up.

3. Sauté onions and mushrooms in butter in a thick bottom pot, until onions and mushrooms turn golden. Season with salt, pepper and thyme.

4. Add cheese, water and wine. Stir. Bring to a boil for a few minutes and then lower the heat to medium and let simmer for 15 minutes.

5. Whisk the heavy cream until soft peaks form. Add yolks and mix well.

6. Fold the egg cream into the soup without boiling it further.

7. Add oil, parsley, salt and pepper in a tall beaker. Use an immersion blender for 30 seconds or until the oil and the parsley are merged together.

8. Serve the soup with a spoonful of parsley oil and prosciutto ham chips on top.

Tip! Regular white wine or one-part white wine vinegar and water gives this creamy soup a nice flavor. You can of course skip wine, then squeeze some lemon juice into the green oil. Also, you can make the soup vegetarian by substituting roasted nuts for the prosciutto chips.

KETO SOUP RECIPES

CAULIFLOWER, LEEK & COCONUT CREAM SOUP

Servings: 4

Nutritional Facts Per Serving:
Net Carbs: 23.8 g   Protein: 3.3 g
Fat: 6.8 g   Calories: 169.5 kcal

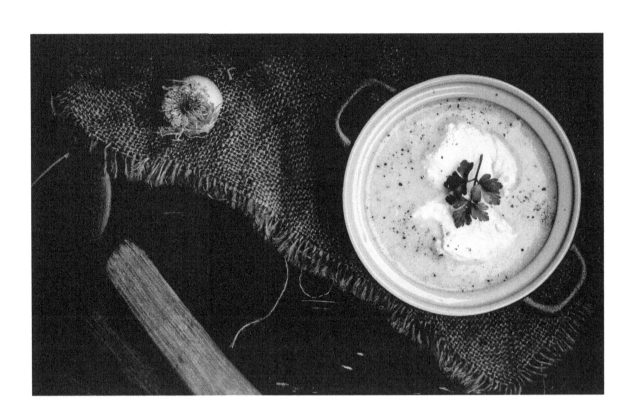

INGREDIENTS

1 large leek
½ cauliflower
½ cup coconut cream, warmed + 2 additional tbsp for drizzling
3 cups chicken or bone broth
Sea salt to taste

This is how you make the recipe

1. Cut the cauliflower and leek into small pieces.

2. Place the cauliflower and leek into a large pot or pressure cooker, then pour in the broth.

3. Cover the pot and simmer for 1 hour or until tender.

4. Use an immersion blender to purée the vegetables to create a smooth soup. (If you don't have an immersion blender, you can take the vegetables out, let cool briefly, purée in a normal blender, and then put back into the pot.)

5. Add in the coconut cream, salt to taste and mix well. Serve and enjoy!

KETO SOUP RECIPES

CREAMY CURRIED CAULIFLOWER SOUP

Servings: 8

Nutritional Facts Per Serving:
Net Carbs: 5.2 g   Protein: 3.5 g
Fat: 14.8 g   Calories: 165 kcal

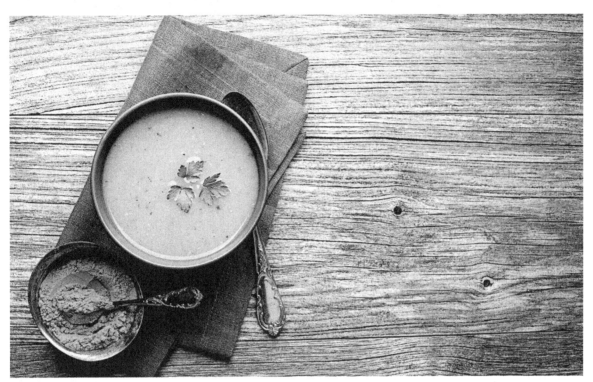

INGREDIENTS

1 large cauliflower, cut into florets
2 tbsp avocado oil or fat of choice
1 white onion, roughly chopped
4 garlic cloves, roughly chopped
1-inch ginger, roughly chopped
½ serrano pepper, seeds removed, roughly chopped
2 tsp curry powder
1 tsp sea salt
½ tsp black pepper
¼ tsp turmeric powder
1 cup filtered water
1 cup chicken or vegetable broth
1 can full-fat coconut milk
Cilantro for garnish (optional)

This is how you make the recipe

1. Add the oil and onions to a Dutch oven or heavy bottomed pot over medium heat and sauté until the onions begin to turn golden brown.

2. Add the garlic, ginger and serrano pepper and stir-fry for 1-2 minutes.

3. Add curry powder, salt, pepper and turmeric.

4. Stir-fry for a minute then add cauliflower florets and 1 cup water.

5. Cover with a lid and cook for 5 minutes – give it a stir – then cook for another 5 minutes or until the cauliflower is soft.

6. Turn off heat, allow the cauliflower to cool – then blend.

7. Pour blended cauliflower back into pot along with broth and coconut milk.

8. Cook for another 5-10 minutes then garnish with cilantro (optional) and serve.

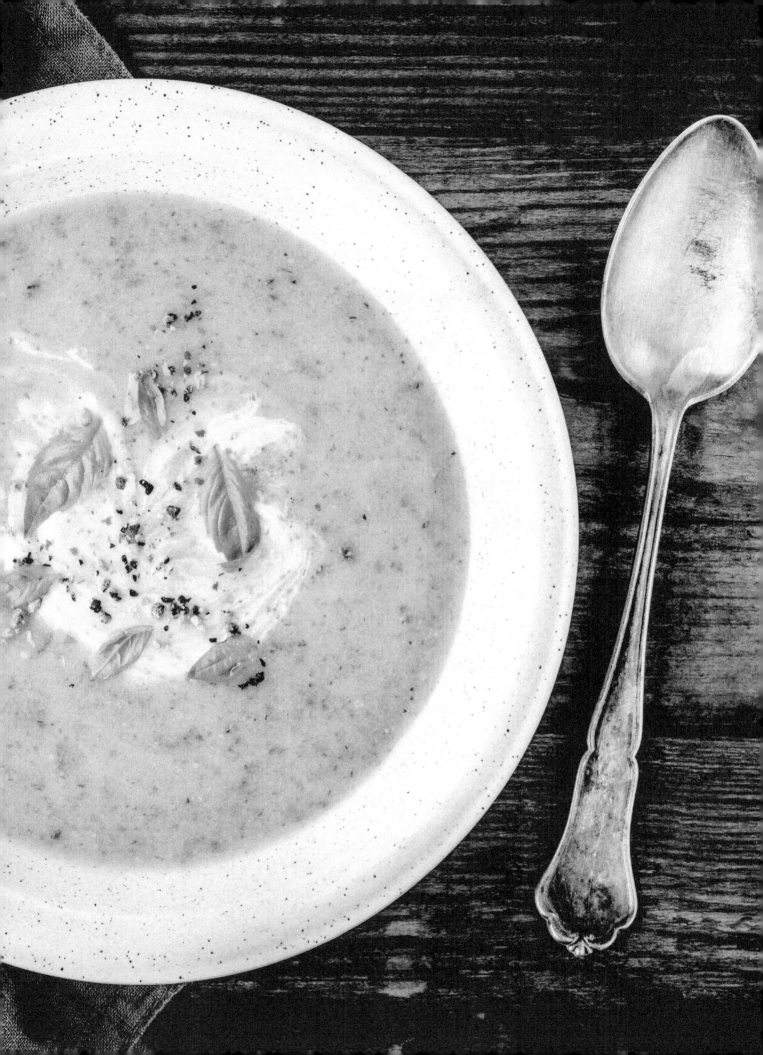

CREAMY BROCCOLI & LEEK SOUP

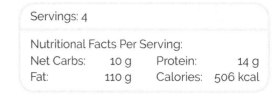

Servings: 4

Nutritional Facts Per Serving:
Net Carbs: 10 g   Protein: 14 g
Fat: 110 g   Calories: 506 kcal

INGREDIENTS

1 leek
1 ¼ cup broccoli
2 cups filtered water
1 vegetable bouillon cube
7 oz cream cheese
1 cup heavy whipping cream
½ tsp black pepper
½ cup fresh basil
1 garlic clove, pressed
Sea salt
Cheese chips:
½ cup cheddar cheese or Edam cheese
½ tsp paprika powder

This is how you make the recipe

1. Broccoli soup: Rinse the leek thoroughly and chop finely, both the green and the white parts. Cut off the core of the broccoli and slice thinly. Divide the rest of the broccoli into smaller florets, and reserve.

2. Place the leek and the sliced broccoli core in a pot and cover with water. Add bouillon cube. Season with salt, and bring to a boil for a few minutes on high heat until the broccoli stem is just easily pierced with a knife.

3. Add the broccoli florets. Lower the heat and simmer for a few minutes, until the broccoli is bright green and tender. Add cream cheese, cream, freshly ground pepper, basil and garlic.

4. Blend with an immersion blender until desired consistency.

5. If the soup is too thick, thin it out with water. If you'd like it to have a slightly thicker consistency, add a touch of heavy cream.

6. Cheese chips: Fit a large, rimmed baking sheet with parchment paper. Grate the cheese, and place mounds by the tbsp on the parchment. Leave 1 inch between the cheese mounds.

7. Top each cheese mound with paprika.

8. Bake in oven at 400°F until the cheese has melted, about 5-6 minutes. Enjoy with a soup or as a snack.

KETO SOUP RECIPES

CREAM OF MUSHROOM SOUP

Servings: 2

Nutritional Facts Per Serving:
Net Carbs: 9.1 g Protein: 6 g
Fat: 4.4 g Calories: 110.5 kcal

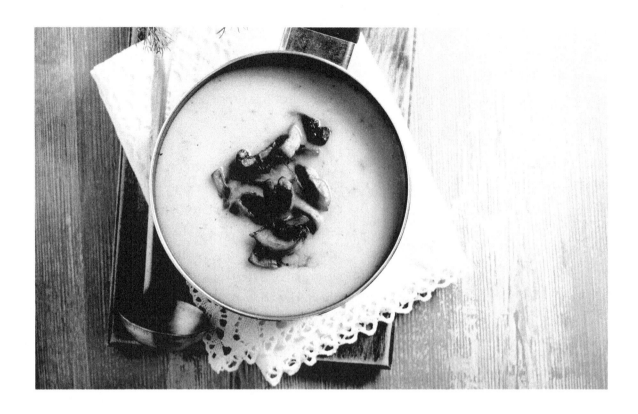

INGREDIENTS

2 cups cauliflower florets
1 ⅔ cup unsweetened original almond milk
1 tsp onion powder
¼ tsp Himalayan salt
Freshly ground pepper, to taste
½ tsp olive oil
1 ½ cups diced white mushrooms
½ yellow onion, diced

This is how you make the recipe

1. Place cauliflower, milk, onion powder, salt and pepper in a small saucepan. Cover and bring to a boil over medium heat. Reduce heat to low and simmer for 7-8 minutes, until cauliflower is softened. Then, purée using a food processor, immersion blender or blender.

2. Meanwhile, add oil, mushrooms and onion to a medium-sized saucepan. Heat over high heat until onions are translucent and beginning to brown, about 8 minutes.

3. Add puréed cauliflower mixture to sautéed mushrooms. Bring to a boil, cover and simmer for 10 minutes, until thickened.

4. Serve immediately and enjoy!

KETO SOUP RECIPES

SHIITAKI MUSHROOM, SPINACH & ASPARAGUS SOUP

Servings: 4

Nutritional Facts Per Serving:
Net Carbs: 18.9 g   Protein: 12.3 g
Fat: 10 g   Calories: 220.3 kcal

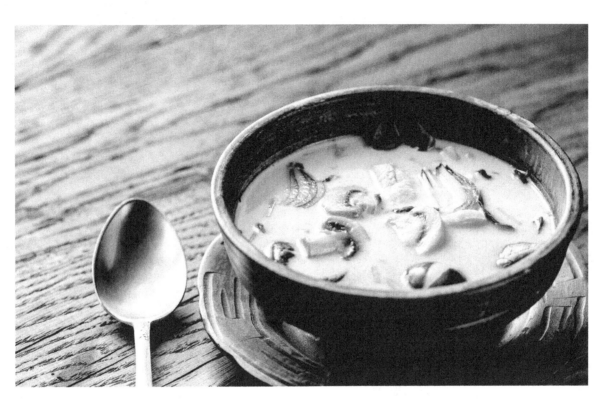

INGREDIENTS

1 lb asparagus, ends trimmed off and cut into ½-inch pieces
2 cups fresh shiitake mushrooms, chopped into thin slices
4 big handfuls of baby spinach, washed well and roughly chopped
1 small onion, finely chopped
4 cloves garlic, minced
4 cups bone or vegetable broth
½ tsp tarragon, dried
1 bay leaf
1 cup nut milk of choice
¼ cup fresh parsley, finely chopped
juice of 1 lemon
Sea salt and black pepper to taste
2 tbsp butter, ghee, or coconut oil

This is how you make the recipe

1. Melt fat of choice in medium soup pot and sauté onion until translucent and beginning to brown.

2. Add minced garlic and sauté for about a minute.

3. Add asparagus and shiitake mushrooms and sauté for 3-4 minutes until they start to sweat.

4. Pour in 4 cups of broth and add bay leaf, tarragon, and spinach.

5. Simmer soup for about 30 minutes on medium-low until asparagus is nice and soft.

6. Turn off heat, add nut milk, lemon juice and fresh parsley, cover and let sit on stove top for at least another 30 minutes. Discard the bay leaf.

7. Add salt and pepper to taste, serve and enjoy!

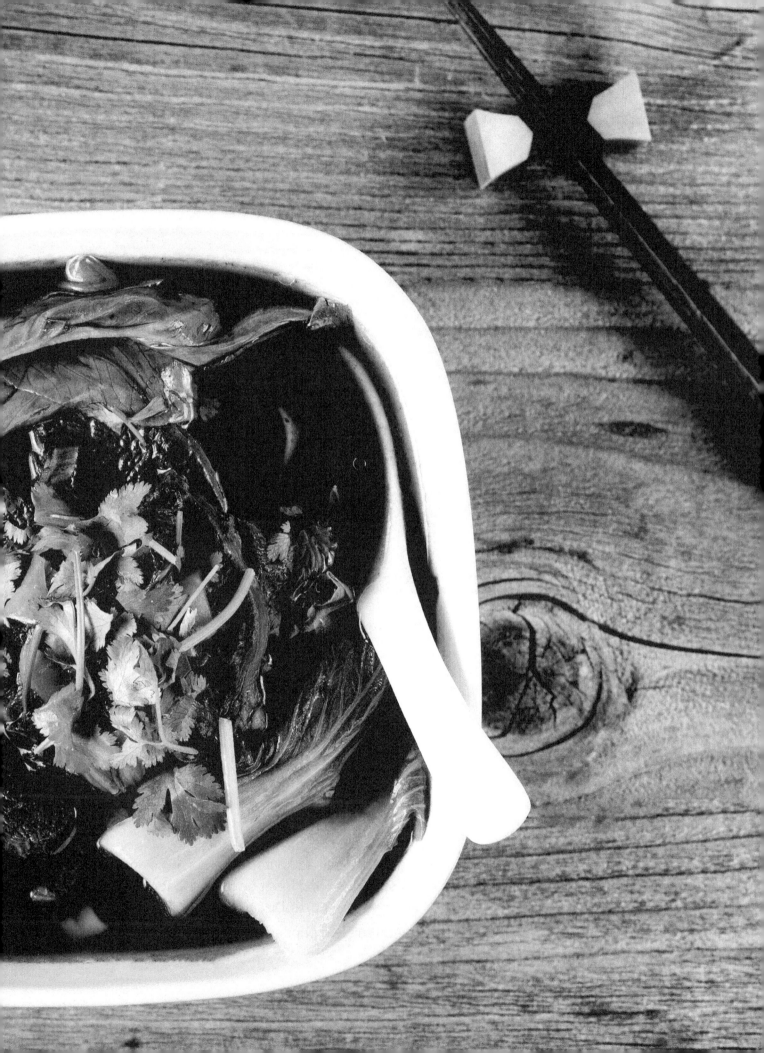

BEEF NOODLE SOUP WITH SHIITAKE MUSHROOMS & BABY BOK CHOY

Servings: 1

Nutritional Facts Per Serving:
Net Carbs: 11.9 g Protein: 30 g
Fat: 41 g Calories: 539 kcal

INGREDIENTS

½ large zucchini, peeled and spiralized
2 tsp minced garlic
3 oz New York strip steak, cut into 1-inch cubes
¼ tsp crushed red pepper flakes
1 ½ tbsp olive oil
¼ cup of water
1 cup chicken broth
1 tbsp coconut aminos
1 head of baby bok choy, roughly chopped (about 3-inch pieces)
½ cup shiitake mushrooms
¼ heaping cup chopped green onions
Sea salt and black pepper to taste

This is how you make the recipe

1. Season the beef cubes with salt, pepper and lightly pat with olive oil.

2. Place a large saucepan over medium heat and add in 1 tbsp of the olive oil.

3. Once the oil heats, add in the garlic.

4. Once the garlic heats, add in the beef and cook for about 1-2 minutes per side or until it is still rare in the middle but seared on the outsides.

5. Remove from the saucepan, leaving in the garlic, and set aside.

6. Place the rest of the olive oil in the same saucepan and add in the red pepper flakes, bok choy and mushrooms. Stir to combine and cook for about 2 minutes.

7. Add in the water and chicken broth and bring to a boil.

8. Once boiled, add in the coconut aminos. Reduce heat and simmer for 5 minutes.

9. Add in the beef, zucchini noodles, and half of the green onions. Cook for 2 minutes and then pour into a bowl.

10. Top with remaining green onions and enjoy!

SIMPLE EGG-DROP SOUP

Servings: 8

Nutritional Facts Per Serving:
Net Carbs: 2 g Protein: 5.9 g
Fat: 1.4 g Calories: 45.5 kcal

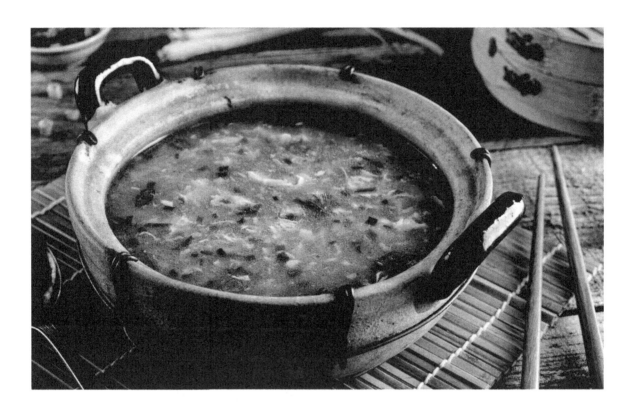

INGREDIENTS

3 cups bone broth
2 cups Swiss chard, chopped
2 eggs, whisked
2 tbsp coconut aminos
1 tsp grated ginger
1 tsp ground oregano
Sea salt and black pepper to taste

This is how you make the recipe

1. Heat up the bone broth in a saucepan.
2. Slowly drizzle in the whisked eggs while stirring slowly clockwise until the ribbons form.
3. Add the Swiss chard, coconut aminos, grated ginger, oregano and salt and pepper, and let it cook for a few minutes.

BACON, LEEK & CAULIFLOWER SOUP

Servings: 4

Nutritional Facts Per Serving:
Net Carbs: 4.7 g
Fat: 6 g
Protein: 8 g
Calories: 108 kcal

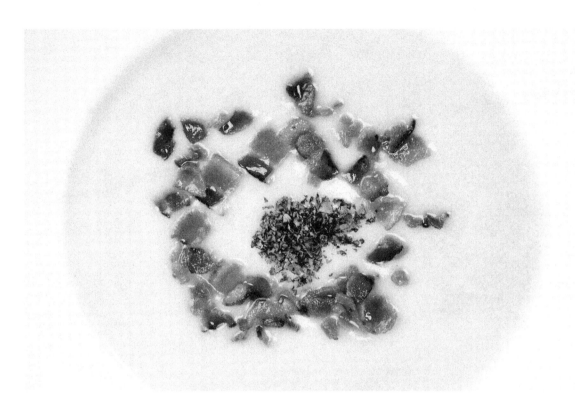

INGREDIENTS

½ head of cauliflower
4 cups of chicken broth or vegetable broth
1 leek
5 strips of bacon
Sea salt and black pepper to taste

This is how you make the recipe

1. Cut the cauliflower and leek into small pieces.
2. Place the cauliflower and leek into the pot with the chicken broth.
3. Boil on medium heat for 1 – 1 ½ hours until tender.
4. Use an immersion blender to purée the vegetables to create a smooth soup. (If you don't have an immersion blender, you can take the vegetables out and purée in a normal blender and then put it back into the pot.)
5. Fry bacon strips until crispy. Cut into small pieces and drop into the soup.
6. Cook on a low heat for 30 minutes.
7. Add salt and pepper to taste.

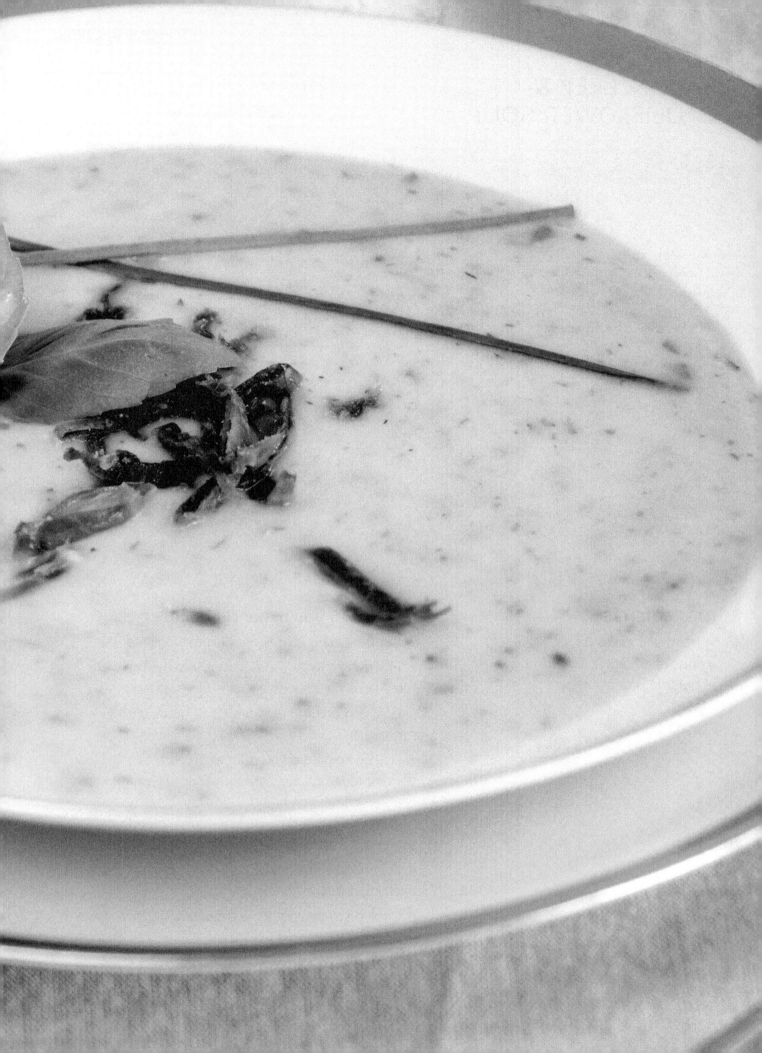

CREAMY PULLED PORK SOUP

Servings: 4

Nutritional Facts Per Serving:
Net Carbs: 22.5 g | Protein: 16.5 g
Fat: 7.25 g | Calories: 232.75 kcal

INGREDIENTS

2 tsp coconut or avocado oil
1 medium onion
8 cloves garlic
1 ½ lb cauliflower
1 tsp sea salt
7 cups chicken or pork broth
2 tsp dried oregano
2 ½ cups pulled pork

This is how you make the recipe

1. Heat a saucepan or Dutch oven over medium-low heat. Dice the onion, then smash and peel the whole garlic cloves. Add the oil, diced onion and smashed garlic to the pan, stirring through the oil to coat. Allow the onion and garlic to soften, stirring occasionally to avoid any burning or coloring.

2. Meanwhile, chop the cauliflower into evenly sized florets and add to the pan along with the salt and broth. Increase the heat to medium-high and bring the broth to a simmer. Cook until the cauliflower is fork tender, about 20 minutes.

3. Remove the pan from the heat and use an immersion blender to blend everything together until you have a smooth, creamy soup base. Add the oregano leaves and return the pan to the heat.

4. Turn the heat to medium and bring the soup back up to a simmer. If the soup is thicker than you prefer, add a little extra broth until the soup is the texture that you like. Add the pulled pork and cook until the pork is hot all the way through before serving.

CHEESY ZUCCHINI SOUP

Servings: 4

Nutritional Facts Per Serving:
Net Carbs: 7.9 g   Protein: 8 g
Fat: 8.5 g   Calories: 140.3 kcal

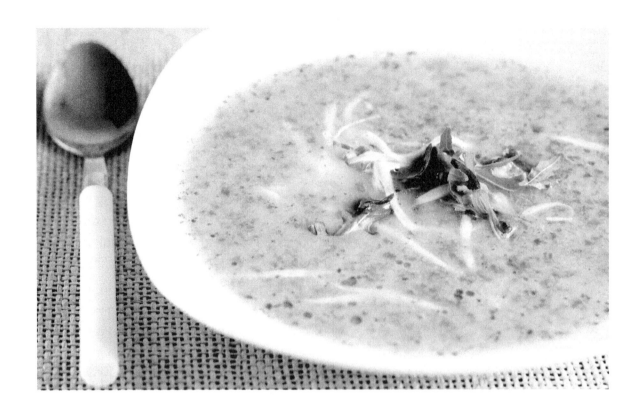

INGREDIENTS

2 tbsp of coconut oil
1 medium onion, peeled and chopped
3 zucchinis, cut into chunks
2 cups bone broth
1 tbsp of nutritional yeast
Pinch of freshly ground black pepper
1 tbsp of coconut cream for garnish
1 tbsp parsley, chopped for garnish

This is how you make the recipe

1. Over medium heat, melt the coconut oil in a large pan. Add the onions and cook until soft.

2. Add the zucchinis and bone broth and reduce to a simmer. Partially cover the pan with a lid and cook until the zucchinis have completely cooked through. They should slide effortlessly off a fork when pierced.

3. Stir in the nutritional yeast and remove the pan from the heat.

4. Use an immersion blender or food processor to blitz the mixture to a fine soup purée.

5. Season with freshly ground black pepper and serve garnished with a decorative drizzle of coconut cream and chopped parsley.

SIMPLE COCONUT SEAFOOD SOUP

KETO SOUP RECIPES

Servings: 4

Nutritional Facts Per Serving:
Net Carbs: 65.3 g Protein: 106.3 g
Fat: 29.5 g Calories: 964.8 kcal

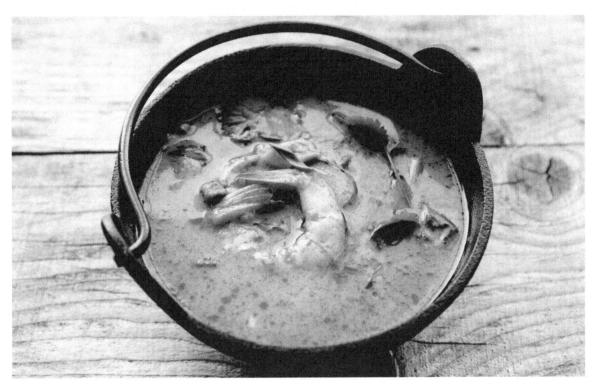

INGREDIENTS

4 cups chicken stock
10 button mushrooms (or other mushrooms), sliced
½ cup kale, chopped
1 cup romaine lettuce, chopped
4 tilapia fillets, chopped into large chunks
10 shrimp/prawns
10 mussels (optional)
1 cup coconut cream
1 tsp Red Boat fish sauce (optional)
Sea salt to taste

This is how you make the recipe

1. Pour the chicken stock into a large pot and bring to a boil.

2. Add in the mushrooms, kale, and romaine lettuce, and bring to a boil again.

3. Add in the tilapia pieces, the shrimp/prawns, and any other seafood, and bring to a boil again. (Ensure the soup covers all the seafood – add in more chicken stock if necessary.)

4. Boil for around 4 minutes until the shrimp/prawns have turned pink and the tilapia pieces are no longer translucent.

5. Add in the coconut cream, fish sauce (optional), and salt to taste. Stir to mix (but be careful not to break up the fish pieces too much).

6. Wait for it to just start boiling, then take off the heat.

7. Serve immediately and enjoy!

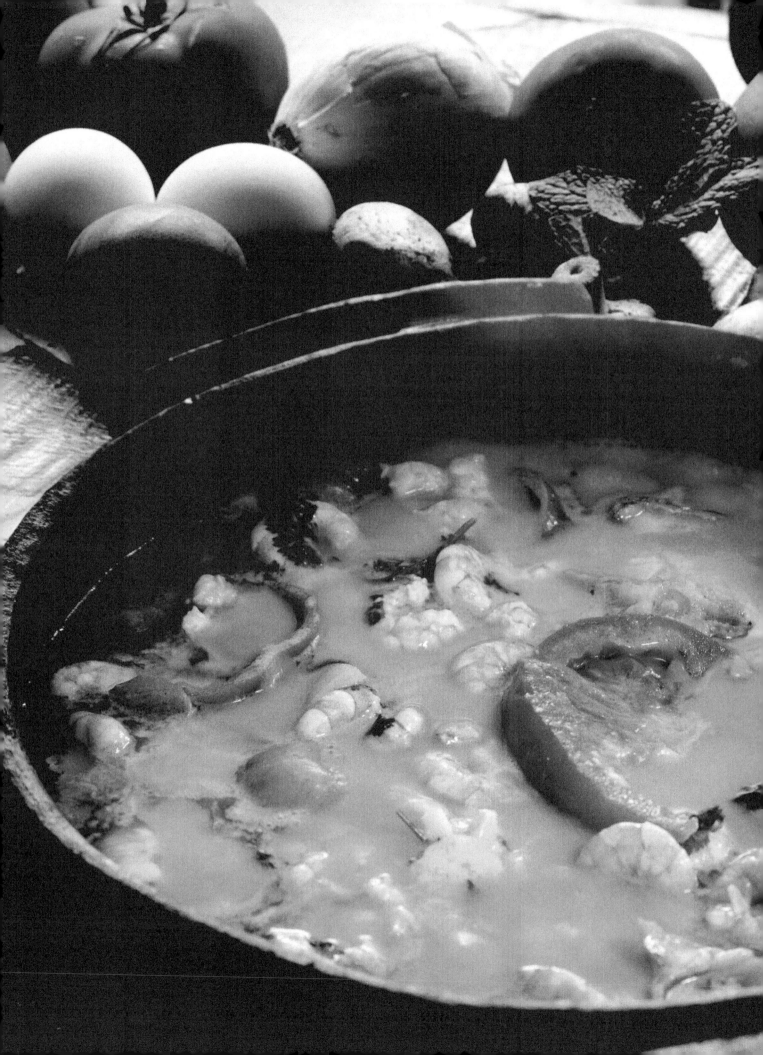

BRAZILIAN HOT SHRIMP SOUP

Servings: 6

Nutritional Facts Per Serving:
Net Carbs: 7.4 g Protein: 17 g
Fat: 18.5 g Calories: 260 kcal

INGREDIENTS

1 ½ lb raw shrimp, peeled & deveined
¼ cup olive oil
¼ cup onion, diced
1 clove garlic, minced
¼ cup roasted red pepper, diced
¼ cup fresh cilantro, chopped
1 (14 oz) can diced tomatoes with chilies
1 cup coconut milk
2 tbsp Sriracha hot sauce
2 tbsp fresh lime juice
Sea salt and black pepper to taste

This is how you make the recipe

1. Heat olive oil in a medium saucepan. Sauté onions for several minutes until translucent, then add the garlic and peppers and cook for several minutes more. Add the tomatoes, shrimp and cilantro to the pan and simmer gently until the shrimp turns opaque. Pour in the coconut milk and Sriracha sauce, and cook just until heated through – do not boil. Add lime juice and season with salt and pepper to taste.

2. Serve hot, garnished with fresh cilantro (optional).

KETO SOUP RECIPES

CREAMY LEEK & SALMON SOUP

Servings: 4

Nutritional Facts Per Serving:
Net Carbs: 11.9 g   Protein: 29.5 g
Fat: 31.3 g   Calories: 444.8 kcal

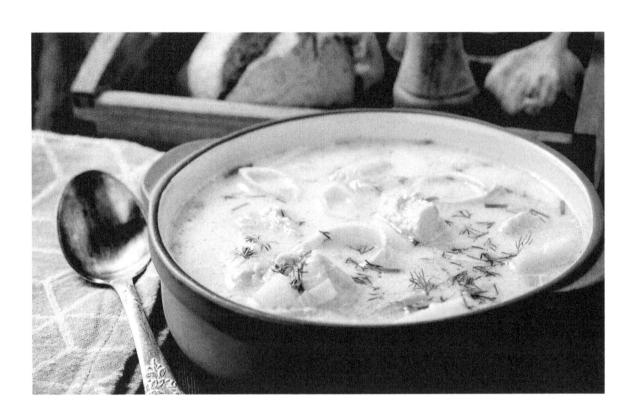

INGREDIENTS

2 tbsp avocado oil
4 leeks, washed, trimmed and sliced into crescents
3 cloves garlic, minced
6 cups seafood or chicken broth
2 tsp dried thyme leaves
1 lb salmon, in bite-size pieces
1 ¾ cup coconut milk
Salt and black pepper to taste

This is how you make the recipe

1. Heat the avocado oil in a large saucepan or Dutch oven at a medium-low heat.

2. Add the chopped leeks and garlic and cook until slightly softened.

3. Pour in the stock and add the thyme. Simmer for about 15 minutes and season to taste with salt and pepper.

4. Add the salmon and the coconut milk to the pan. Bring back up to a gentle simmer and cook until the fish is opaque and tender.

5. Serve immediately and enjoy!

SALMON SOUP

Servings: 4

Nutritional Facts Per Serving:
Net Carbs: 8.7 g   Protein: 46.5 g
Fat: 24.5 g   Calories: 459.3 kcal

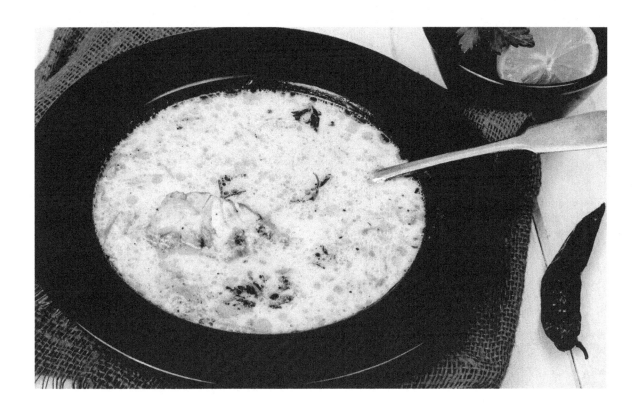

INGREDIENTS

4 cups chicken broth
1½ lb salmon fillets
1 cup parsley, chopped
3 cups Swiss chard or spinach or cavalo nero, roughly chopped
2 Italian squash, chopped
1 clove of garlic, crushed
Juice from ½ a lemon
Sea salt and black pepper to taste
2 eggs (optional)

This is how you make the recipe

1. Pour the chicken broth into a pot and start heating it up.

2. While the broth is heating up, chop the vegetables and drop them along with the crushed garlic into the pot.

3. Then chop up the salmon into strips or chunks and drop into the pot.

4. Add the lemon juice.

5. Cook for 10 minutes on a medium heat.

6. Crack 2 eggs into the pot and stir it up (make sure to break the yolk).

7. Add salt and pepper to taste.

8. Serve and enjoy!

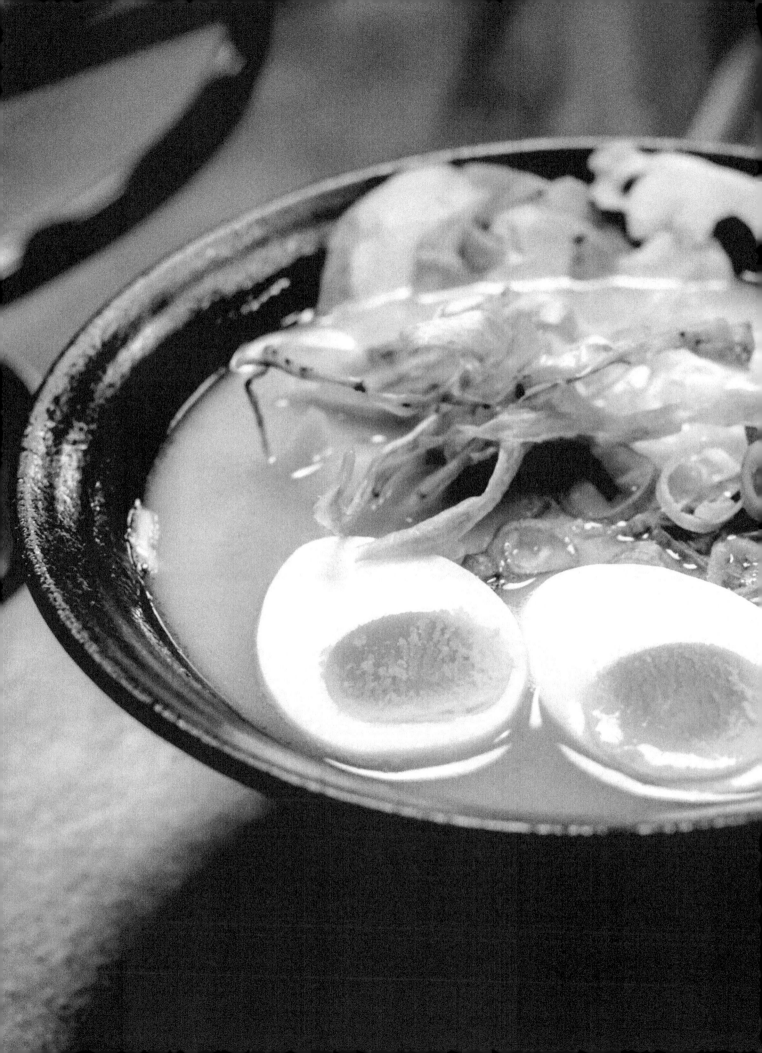

CHICKEN SOUP

Servings: 2

Nutritional Facts Per Serving:
Net Carbs: 6.9 g Protein: 31.5 g
Fat: 29.5 g Calories: 421 kcal

INGREDIENTS

1 chicken breast, sliced
4 cups chicken broth
2 eggs
1 zucchini, made into noodles
1 tbsp ginger, minced
2 cloves of garlic, peeled and minced
2 tbsp gluten-free tamari sauce or coconut aminos
3 tbsp avocado oil

This is how you make the recipe

1. Pan-fry the chicken slices in the avocado oil in a large frying pan until cooked and browned.

2. Hard boil the 2 eggs and slice in half.

3. Add chicken broth to a large pot and simmer with the ginger, garlic, tamari sauce, and add in the zucchini noodles for 2-3 minutes to soften them.

4. Divide the broth into 2 bowls, top with the boiled eggs and chicken breast slices.

5. Season with additional hot sauce or tamari sauce, to taste.

KETO SOUP RECIPES

THAI CHICKEN BROTH

Servings: 10

Nutritional Facts Per Serving:
Net Carbs: 0.9 g Protein: 16.4 g
Fat: 8.2 g Calories: 147 kcal

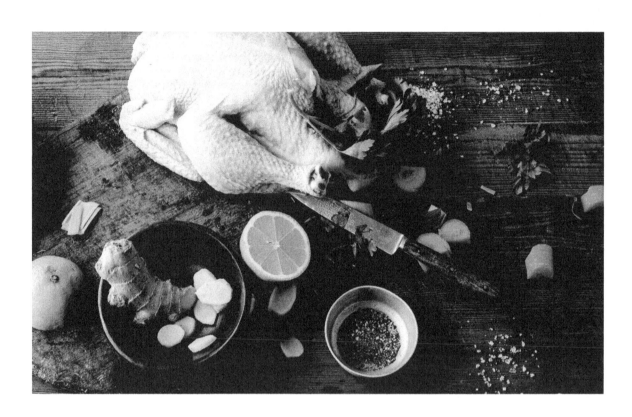

INGREDIENTS

1 whole chicken
1 stalk of lemongrass, cut into large chunks
20 fresh basil leaves (10 for the slow cooker, and 10 for garnish)
5 thick slices of fresh ginger
1 lime
1 tbsp sea salt, or more, to taste

This is how you make the recipe

1. Place the chicken, lemongrass, 10 basil leaves, ginger, and salt into the slow cooker.

2. Fill up the slow cooker with water.

3. Cook on low for 8-10 hours.

4. Ladle the broth into a bowl, add in salt to taste, squeeze in fresh lime juice to taste, and garnish with chopped basil leaves.

5. Serve and enjoy!

KETO SOUP RECIPES

ENCHILADA CHICKEN SOUP

Servings: 4

Nutritional Facts Per Serving:
Net Carbs: 7.6 g   Protein: 40.8 g
Fat: 12.8 g   Calories: 325.3 kcal

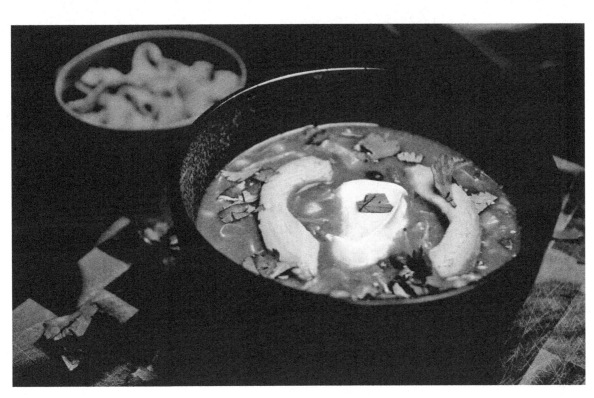

INGREDIENTS

2 tsp of olive oil
1 red onion
2 tsp of cumin powder
1 tsp of cayenne pepper
2 cloves of garlic, peeled and finely chopped
4 chicken breasts, skinless
2 tsp of dried oregano
3 ½ cups of chicken broth
10 oz of diced tomatoes
1 yellow bell pepper, chopped
Sea salt and pepper to taste
2 slices tomato, halved for garnish
1 large avocado, diced for garnish
Cilantro, finely chopped for garnish
½ red chili pepper, seeds removed and finely chopped for garnish

This is how you make the recipe

1. Finely chop the red onion and set aside 2 tbsp to use as garnish.

2. Cook onions in a pan with olive oil until soft and caramelized. Halfway through, add the cumin, cayenne pepper, and garlic.

3. Add the onions, chicken, and oregano to the slow cooker. Pour in the chicken broth and tomatoes. Cover and cook for on high for 2 ½ hours.

4. Add the bell pepper and cook for another 30 minutes.

5. Shred the chicken. Season with salt and pepper.

6. Garnish with a small slice tomato, avocado, cilantro, red chili, and onions.

7. Serve and enjoy!

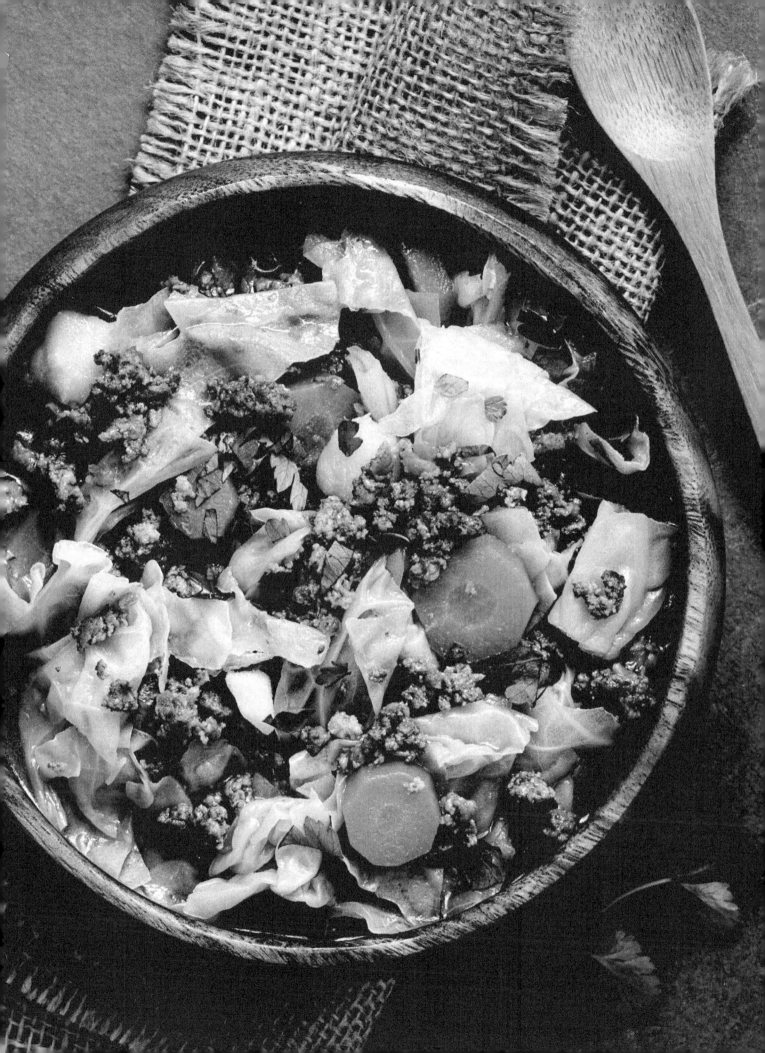

CABBAGE SOUP

Servings: 10

Nutritional Facts Per Serving:
Net Carbs: 6.7 g   Protein: 26.7 g
Fat: 16.1 g   Calories: 288.5 kcal

INGREDIENTS

2 lb ground beef
¼ large onion, diced
1 clove garlic, minced
1 tsp cumin, ground
1 head cabbage large, chopped
4 cubes bouillon
1 can Ro-tel
4 cups filtered water
Sea salt and black pepper to taste

This is how you make the recipe

1. Brown ground beef over medium heat. Add onion and cook until translucent.

2. Transfer ground beef and onion mixture to stock pot.

3. Add garlic, cumin, cabbage, bouillon cubes, Ro-tel and water to the stock pot.

4. Mix ingredients thoroughly and bring to a boil over high heat.

5. Reduce heat to medium-low and simmer covered for 30 - 45 minutes.

6. Serve and enjoy!

KETO SOUP RECIPES

THAI BEEF & BROCCOLI SOUP

Servings: 6

Nutritional Facts Per Serving:
Net Carbs: 9.8 g   Protein: 30 g
Fat: 26.5 g   Calories: 404 kcal

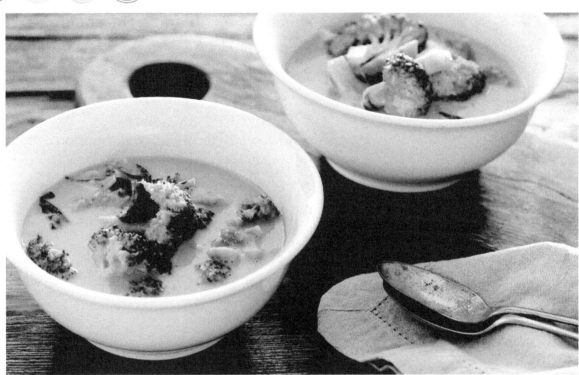

INGREDIENTS

2 tbsp avocado oil or fat of choice
1 onion, chopped
2 tbsp Thai green curry paste, adjust to taste
2-inch knob ginger, minced
2 garlic cloves, minced
1 serrano pepper, minced
1 lb ground beef
3 tbsp coconut aminos
2 tsp fish sauce
½ tsp sea salt
½ tsp black pepper
4 cups beef bone broth or chicken stock
2 large stalks of broccoli, cut into florets
1 cup of full-fat canned coconut milk
Cilantro for garnish

This is how you make the recipe

1. Add the oil and onions to a Dutch oven and cook for 10 minutes, or until the onions begin to turn golden.

2. Add the curry paste, ginger, garlic and serrano pepper and stir for a minute.

3. Next, add the ground beef, coconut aminos, fish sauce, salt and pepper and cook until the beef is nearly brown.

4. Add the broth, reduce the heat to medium-low. Cover the pot with a lid and cook for 20 minutes.

5. Add the broccoli florets and coconut milk to the pot, cover and cook for another 10 minutes.

6. Remove the lid, increase heat to high and simmer for 5 minutes.

7. Garnish with cilantro, serve and enjoy!

Made in the USA
Coppell, TX
03 January 2020